Register Now for Online Access to Your Book!

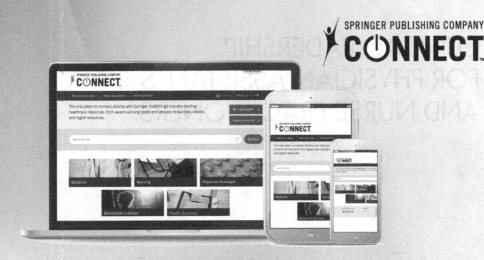

CLINICAL LEADERSHIP FOR PHYSICIAN ASSISTANTS AND NURSE PRACTITIONERS

Michael J. Huckabee, PhD, MPAS, PA-C, is the founding director of the Mayo Clinic Physician Assistant Program and associate professor in the Mayo Clinic College of Medicine and Science. He has over 35 years of clinical practice as a physician assistant (PA), primarily in rural Nebraska. Dr. Huckabee has served as director of PA education at the University of Nebraska Medical Center in Omaha and Union College in Lincoln, Nebraska, and prior to that was a faculty member at the University of Iowa in Iowa City. Over the course of his career, he has managed federally funded projects nearing $3 million that continue to support healthcare for underserved populations. Dr. Huckabee is widely published on several healthcare and educational subjects and is well known in the leadership field, speaking at conferences on topics such as effective leadership strategies and influencing progress by servant leadership. Dr. Huckabee is a Fellow of the American Academy of Physician Assistants and has served as Abstracts and Brief Reports editor for the *Journal of Physician Assistant Education.*

CLINICAL LEADERSHIP FOR PHYSICIAN ASSISTANTS AND NURSE PRACTITIONERS

Michael J. Huckabee, PhD, MPAS, PA-C

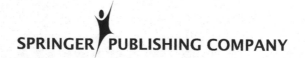

SPRINGER PUBLISHING COMPANY

Springer Publishing Company, LLC
11 West 42nd Street
New York, NY 10036
www.springerpub.com

Acquisitions Editor: Suzanne Toppy
Compositor: S4Carlisle Publishing Services

ISBN: 978-0-8261-7221-1
ebook ISBN: 978-0-8261-7222-8
Instructor's Worksheets ISBN: 978-0-8261-7223-5

Instructor's Materials: Qualified instructors may request supplements by emailing textbook@springerpub.com

17 18 19 20/5 4 3 2 1

The author and the publisher of this Work have made every effort to use sources believed to be reliable to provide information that is accurate and compatible with the standards generally accepted at the time of publication. Because medical science is continually advancing, our knowledge base continues to expand. Therefore, as new information becomes available, changes in procedures become necessary. We recommend that the reader always consult current research and specific institutional policies before performing any clinical procedure. The author and publisher shall not be liable for any special, consequential, or exemplary damages resulting, in whole or in part, from the readers' use of, or reliance on, the information contained in this book. The publisher has no responsibility for the persistence or accuracy of URLs for external or third-party Internet websites referred to in this publication and does not guarantee that any content on such websites is, or will remain, accurate or appropriate.

Library of Congress Cataloging-in-Publication Data

Names: Huckabee, Michael Joseph, author.
Title: Clinical leadership for physician assistants and nurse practitioners /
    Michael J. Huckabee.
Description: New York : Springer Publishing Company, [2018] | Includes
    bibliographical references and index.
Identifiers: LCCN 2017037025| ISBN 9780826172211 | ISBN 9780826172235
    (instructor's worksheets) | ISBN 9780826172228 (e-book)
Subjects: | MESH: Leadership | Physician Assistants | Nurse Practitioners
Classification: LCC R697.P45 | NLM W 21.5 | DDC 610.73/7069--dc23 LC record available at
https://lccn.loc.gov/2017037025

Printed in the United States of America by Gasch Printing.

CONTENTS

FOREWORD

It is a great honor and privilege to have been asked to introduce this valuable book, *Clinical Leadership for Physician Assistants and Nurse Practitioners*—a book that offers a most welcome guide to those who aspire to lead health care now and into the future. As a nurse, I fully endorse a key tenet of the Institute of Medicine's (IOM's) report, *The Future of Nursing: Leading Change, Advancing Health* (IOM, 2011), that "Nurses should be full partners, with physicians, and other health professionals, in redesigning health care in the United States" (p. 8). This means interprofessional partnership and collaboration at every level of the current and future health care system—including among advanced practice providers (APPs).

Our new health care environment is rapidly changing and demanding better care for individuals, improved health outcomes for populations, and lower costs for consumers. In this new environment of rapid change and increasing complexity, health care professionals are being challenged to lead health care systems that offer universal accessibility, coordination across all points of care, and the delivery of high-quality, safe care—and all this at an affordable price. This environment challenges leaders in health care to understand and embrace collaboration, team-based care, and partnerships, and to focus on providing excellence for health care consumers in achieving optimal health outcomes (Salmond & Forrester, 2016).

Informed by the historical underpinnings of clinical leadership of APPs—physician assistants (PAs) and nurse practitioners (NPs)—and recognizing the unique attributes of each, this book provides both health professional students and experienced practitioners with the cognitive strategies for clinical leadership and opportunities for applying these strategies to the realities of advanced clinical practice. It offers APPs a clear focus on clinical leadership while providing an important differentiation between true leadership skills and behaviors and mere task-oriented management skills. This is an essential distinction if leadership traits are to be understood, leadership skills are to be attained, and exemplary leadership behaviors are to be manifest. Here, leadership is conceptualized as being concerned with the clinical leader's ability to influence others to achieve specific goals in order to achieve excellence in health care.

This book reports on various leadership theories/models and uses meaningful leadership research evidence that relates well to real-world clinical settings while cautioning the reader to understand that research findings may not always produce predictable leadership outcomes, owing to the complexities inherent in today's complex clinical practice environment. Administrative leadership strategies are explicated for PAs and NPs, vis-à-vis the financial principles of clinical leadership and change strategies used by clinical leaders to achieve desired, planned change in complex health care environments. Human aspects of clinical leadership are rarely addressed in health professionals' literature but are certainly included here—the importance of clinical leaders being ethical and culturally informed in their advanced practice; the potential for and qualities of being a spiritual leader in a clinical setting; teaching others and leading other leaders in a clinical setting; and resiliency of the clinical leader in preventing burnout. Finally, this book invites readers to look ahead to the future and ponder the possibilities of a desired future for health care.

This much-needed book is an excellent resource for the next generation of leaders in health care. It is my hope that this book will educate, inspire, and empower its readers to lead health, health care, and society into a better, healthier future.

David Anthony (Tony) Forrester, PhD, RN, ANEF, FAAN
Professor, Division of Nursing Science,
Rutgers University School of Nursing
Clinical Professor, Rutgers University
Robert Wood Johnson Medical School
Newark, New Jersey

REFERENCES

Institute of Medicine. (2011). *The future of nursing: Leading change, advancing health*. Washington, DC: National Academies Press.

Salmond, S. W., & Forrester, D. A. (2016). Nurses leading change: The time is now! In D. A. Forrester (Ed.), *Nursing's greatest leaders: A history of activism* (pp. 269–286). New York, NY: Springer Publishing.

PREFACE

Words matter.

It may be that nurse practitioners (NPs) and physician assistants (PAs) understand that better than most. Those words describe the identity of each profession. Yet, their professional titles have been misinterpreted and confused since the birth of each occupation. From state and national legislative debate to mainstream marketing, great and costly effort has been made by each profession to communicate the distinguishing qualities that separately define PAs and NPs. The success of these efforts in forging distinct identities remains unclear. Here presents a book that combines the two.

It is reasonable to question why.

Each profession's own history of alternative titles speaks to the dilemma of defining their respective professional identities (see Table P.1). For NPs, questions are raised when distinguishing between the advanced practice registered nurse (APRN), advanced practice nurse (APN), or clinical nurse specialist (CNS). Each title carries its own characteristics, sometimes broadened to identify the specialty of clinical training (e.g., pediatric nurse practitioner [PNP] and women's health nurse practitioner [WHNP]). In addition, NPs, while thankful for the extraordinary heritage of nursing, continue to defend their roles as something beyond traditions widely interpreted by the word *nurse*.

For PAs, it has been recurring internal and marketplace debates to replace the *assistant* word in the physician assistant title, as that word implies a subjugation of the responsibility the PA holds. Physician associate (the term used in the United Kingdom for this professional role) and Medex ("medical extender" in short) took root in some parts of the United States during past attempts to distinguish the PA profession from some type of an apprenticeship. The annoying grammatical error of using an apostrophe

TABLE P.1 Alternative Terms for Nurse Practitioners and Physician Assistants

Physician Assistant	Nurse Practitioner	Inclusive of Both NPs and PAs
Physician associate	Advanced practice RN	Nonphysician providers
Medex	Advanced practice nurse	Mid-level providers
Physician extenders	Clinical nurse specialist	Advanced practice providers*

NP, nurse practitioner; PA, physician assistant; RN, registered nurse.
*Preferred in this book.

"s" (*physician's* assistant), suggesting some type of possessive ownership, remains the bane of the PA.

If one could go back to the beginning, many of these professionals would suggest a different name to better define their identities. Over time and experience, each profession's title, redefined when needed, now reflects its respective professional identity. Here is each profession's definition, using its own words from its respective national professional association.

PHYSICIAN ASSISTANT

A PA is a nationally certified and state-licensed medical professional. PAs practice medicine on health care teams with physicians and other providers. They practice and prescribe medication in all 50 states, the District of Columbia, U.S. territories, and the uniformed services (American Academy of Physician Assistants, https://www.aapa.org/what-is-a-pa).

NURSE PRACTITIONER

Nurse practitioners (NPs) have been providing primary, acute, and specialty health care to patients of all ages and walks of life for nearly half a century. NPs assess patients, order and interpret diagnostic tests, make diagnoses, and initiate and manage treatment plans—including prescribing medications. They are the health care providers of choice for millions of patients (American Association of Nurse Practitioners^{tm}, 2017, www.aanp.org/about-aanp).

Should PAs and NPs Be Combined?

One cannot argue the similarity of the roles of NPs and PAs as they provide robust health care to countless patients. Their respective definitions offer small distinctions, and each profession well knows that by education and professional pursuits there are differences. That does not change the fact that on a day-to-day basis, the practice patterns of the professions overlap. For that reason, many have recommended a title to combine the two professions. "Physician extenders" has been tried, and "nonphysician providers" (NPPs) is used in some research articles and governmental publications. It's not uncommon for the word "clinician" to take the place of "provider" in all terms of this type (e.g., "nonphysician clinicians" [NPCs]). Other health careers brought into the classification to be more inclusive (e.g., nurse anesthetists and nurse midwives) created more challenges when attempting to clarify roles.

The most popular term, *mid-level providers*, required clarification on the intention of the words. Those outside the professions needed to be reminded that in the education, training, and experience of PA and NP clinicians, educators, and researchers, there was no evidence that the duties or practice of either profession were *average* ("mid") or fit in the middle of a continuum from high-level to low-level care. Larger hospitals and health care organizations that employ NPs and PAs are now using the title *advanced practice providers* (or advanced practice professionals [APPs]) for administrative purposes, which has generally been accepted well.

Most from each profession find the greatest satisfaction in using the original titles of PA and NP. The need for a joint title is not necessary as identities are established and generally respected for each profession.

APP Leadership

Building on the strength of each profession's identity, the call for leadership has never been clearer. With full respect for the unique aspects of their respective educational and professional pursuits, the leadership concepts and applications for NPs and PAs are typically quite similar, if not identical. Chapter 1 presents the case for why leadership skills are critical for both professions. For the purposes of this book, exploring leadership in the context of the operational responsibilities of PAs and NPs together offers a relevant and timely discussion.

For convention, when the terms *NP* and *PA* are used together, the order will alternate, similar to varying the order of the words *her and his*, to avoid any indication of preference or priority.

In this book, leadership scenarios specific to each profession strive to distinguish unique features if indicated. When the leadership concepts apply equally to both professions, the term *advanced practice provider* (APP) is used.

LEARNER HELPS

Written both for learners new to the APP professions and for learners with years of experience as PAs or NPs, the reader may find the use of *advance organizers* helpful. These appear as questions at the beginning of each chapter, framed from a learning objective. Each question (advance organizer) poses a cognitive strategy to guide the application and retention of the chapter's content, helping the learner integrate information into practice. Case studies and exercises embedded throughout the book provide additional opportunities for application and practice. Additional learning activities are found in the appendices. **Qualified instructors may obtain access to ancillary instructor's worksheets by emailing textbook@springerpub.com.**

LEADING OPTIMAL HEALTH

With this understanding of the two professions, NPs and PAs, may this book serve to inspire the reader to greater opportunities and success in leadership. The health care delivery systems and, more importantly, the patients receiving care need the APPs' help to influence optimal health outcomes.

Michael J. Huckabee

PART 1
Clinical Leadership Traits and Behaviors

1

WHY CLINICAL LEADERSHIP?

CRITICAL THINKING QUESTIONS

» **What is the definition of leadership in the clinical paradigm of physician assistants (PAs) and nurse practitioners (NPs)?**

» **If advanced practice providers (APPs) do not have ultimate authority, how are they able to function in leadership roles?**

» **What are the distinctions between clinical leaders and clinical managers?**

» **Isn't leadership something innate that some people naturally have and some do not?**

» **How can behavioral research on leadership be helpful when it is vague and less precise than traditional clinical research?**

CASE STUDY 1

As an M3, I was aghast when Dr. Thompson marched us all into Mrs. Banner's room on morning rounds with the Critical Care Team. At her bedside, he shook her hand and opened her gown to auscultate her chest without washing his hands first. My eyes darted to the residents who were clearly nervous. Someone needed to say something. They were next in line to inspect her postop wounds, palpate her abdomen, or otherwise examine her. Who wanted to call out Dr. Thompson on his obvious gaffe in handwashing? I wasn't about to.

Just then, Susan, the PA with Dr. Thompson, casually went to the sidewall dispenser and squirted alcohol cleanser in her hands. She came alongside Dr. Thompson, still rubbing the gel across her hands. "Dr. Thompson, would you like me to check her surgical site?" Immediately, the residents lined up at the Purell dispenser and Dr. Thompson gestured to Susan to continue the examination as he stepped back, still in control, having escaped embarrassment.

EVOLVING HIERARCHIES OF CLINICAL LEADERSHIP

The traditional view of leadership as a hierarchical position of power is fading in the face of other models that are often more effective. The Petri dish of the clinical environment becomes an excellent medium, providing an opportunity to examine best practices. The leadership design in historical medicine placed the physician at the highest position, nurses falling next in order, followed by a scattering of other health care members included at the whim of the physician.

Today's evolving health care environment disrupts this top-down hierarchy by a host of add-ins, whether it be the forces of payers, governmental requirements, administrative directives, or particularly skilled team members who bring a level of expertise to the ever-expanding advancements and technologies of health care.

Enter the APP, typically a PA or NP, who shows by example and action that gains are made in team dynamics, workload balance, patient satisfaction, fiscal bottom-lines, and clinical outcomes. The opening Case Study 1 in this chapter portrays how the PA is able to navigate a difficult situation of the physician's oversight of the need for handwashing prior to patient contact. Here, Susan was able to take action to correct the physician's lapse, delivering the standard quality of care expected by the team and avoiding awkward confrontations or embarrassment of any team members.

Certainly, this success comes from a well-educated individual able to use her or his talents and skills in the midst of a progressive structure. However, not one of these gains could be achieved without an effective health care team that includes individuals who understand their own roles and the roles of those around them. This can happen intuitively, sometimes with success and sometimes without. However, what if the NPs and PAs on the health care team were specifically trained in their respective roles? Instead of hoping for a good blend of personalities so that everyone gets along, those APPs come to the table with a clear understanding of leadership dynamics, skilled in working in, if not managing, teams.

DEFINING LEADERSHIP

In meeting this obligation, a clear focus on leadership skills is necessary. While definitions abound with rich verbiage suited for diverse environments, this text will focus on leadership as *the ability to influence others toward achieving a specific goal*. Three distinct components are included in this definition: (a) the ability to influence, (b) others, and (c) achieving a specific goal.

The Ability to Influence

Influencing others is not dependent on a position of power or authority. The ability to influence includes the opportunity to explore the art of persuasion apart from the forces of coercion. It also requires a dyad that considers those on the receiving end of being influenced, hence the next component of this definition of leadership.

Somewhat unique to the APP role compared to other members of the health care team, the direction of influence is both upward and downward. The APP often makes independent health care decisions for patient care. These decisions bring opportunities for the APP to influence those who will then carry out responsibilities or directives. Examples include the APP directing a patient on the use of provided samples of prescription medication, the NP asking a nutritionist to manage the diet of a patient admitted for heart failure, or a PA ordering imaging examinations to help determine a patient diagnosis.

The upward direction of the APP's ability to influence is often expected by the physician or manager of the clinical services. Some may consider this participative leadership, defined as the leader delegating certain leadership decisions to a member of the team. While this may occur, more often the APP is positioned to influence upward in shaping the direction of the team, including being welcome to contribute contrary thinking to those holding higher authority. APPs, by their position, have the ability to influence upward by, for example, proposing enhanced administrative processes to hospital administrators and respectfully communicating with physicians to modify previous decisions in patient care plans. These and other opportunities for upward influence are common to the NP and PA; those who employ APPs typically anticipate this direction of influence with optimism. New leadership models such as this are replacing the traditional hierarchy of a physician-led health care team as a more effective model of best practice. The ultimate authority for patient care delivery remains in place with the physician or another top-down administrative structure, and the APP within this structure influences the team members upward and downward to achieve the best outcomes.

Others

Peter Drucker, a brilliant mind who has shaped the world of modern management, famously simplified a leader as "someone who has followers" (1996). While this definition deserves expansion tailored to the situation, one must never neglect the truth that a person can lead only if there is someone willing to follow. The attributes and efforts of the follower either make for success or bring failure, so critical attention must be given to the needs and roles of followers.

Understanding the distinctive role of the APP in the health care team with impact upward and downward leaves a broad scope of individuals who can be influenced. In the tight hierarchy of physician – APP – nurse – patient, there are bidirectional opportunities for influence by all members. However, the APP is positioned mid-stream in the flow of the health care organizations to directly influence others on the team. This includes all levels of health care administrative management, hospital committees, state and federal health policy, public health measures, finance, third-party reimbursement, safety, custodial and plant services. These are in addition to those contributing directly to individual patient care such as medical imaging and laboratory, physical and occupational therapies, pathology services, other allied health professionals, and a host of nursing services.

Achieving a Specific Goal

Attuned to the scientific process that guides all of medicine, there must be a measurable outcome as evidence of success. Without intentional direction, both leader and follower wander without aim. Leadership must be goal-directed with clarity and purpose. There are clinical environs that may seek to slow the pace of progress, thankful to have somehow survived an economic crisis. Perhaps the pursuit of a goal is halted because a team faces an expectation that demise, perhaps death, is inevitable. However, like the body's need to maintain blood flow or risk a thrombus that disrupts downstream, a team without purpose may create more problems. Leadership takes the reins to guide through such struggles to a better place.

In the clinical positions of APPs, there are diverse leadership roles. Often these become assumed by default, and kudos to the APP who is willing to carry the responsibility of leadership. Here are examples of leadership roles common to APPs that incorporate the definition of influencing others toward achieving a specific goal:

» Influencing a patient to change lifestyle behaviors for better health (smoking cessation, increased compliance in monitoring blood sugars, etc.)

» Making decisions about immediate nursing care needs in clinic or hospital settings

» As the first assistant in surgical procedures, opening and/or closing surgical sites, providing preop or postop care decisions

» Overseeing targeted health education of patients such as organizing a weekly asthma clinic

» Serving on or chairing health care committees for quality control, infection control, pharmaceutical requirements, ethics, and medical staff policies, among others

» Taking administrative roles that oversee the work of other APPs, nursing and allied health providers

» Conducting health and wellness programs in local communities

» Mentoring future professionals as a preceptor for health professions students

» Owning a health care clinic that serves otherwise underserved patient populations

» Chairing committees or being elected to office in local, state, and national professional organizations such as the American Academy of Physician Assistants, the American Association of Nurse Practitioners, or other professional specialty organizations

» Guiding health care policies or legislative bills through appropriate approval processes

» Holding offices in local, state, and national health organizations such as the American Heart Association and the American Cancer Society

While this list is by no means comprehensive, it gives evidence to the common and effective utilization of APPs. Rather than waiting for leadership responsibilities to arise either by hopeful volunteerism or by crisis, the thoughtful positioning of APP leadership responsibilities will naturally bring a better yield in achieving the specific goals.

LEADERSHIP VERSUS MANAGEMENT

Leadership is most commonly confused with managerial responsibilities. While a leader often carries the tasks of a manager, the role of leadership must maintain preeminence. If a leader's time and thoughts are consumed with management tasks, the ability to influence others toward achieving a specific goal is directly diminished. Common management tasks assumed by the APP may include the following:

» Arranging work/call schedules

» Collecting data on clinical outcomes

» Training others in clinical skills

» Preparing/managing budgets

» Sorting lab results

» Making callbacks

While each of these tasks may serve an important role for which the APP was hired, the responsibilities may detract from the opportunity to lead. If the APP is performing three or more of these types of tasks on a regular basis, she or he is likely not able to give the most effective attention to influencing others toward achieving a specific goal.

To more clearly distinguish between leaders and managers, Table 1.1 offers contrasts in the responsibilities between these two roles. For example, the PA manager would be the one tasked with ensuring a patient is

TABLE 1.1 Distinctions Between Leadership and Management

Leadership	Management
Innovation	Order
New directions	Efficiency
Tolerance of ambiguity	Stability
Priority consensus	Getting things done
Doing the right thing*	Doing things the right way*
Visioning	Action plans
Growth/Expansion	Organizing/Staffing
Creating new standards	Analyzing results

*Bennis and Nanus (1985).

prepared for surgery with charted and reviewed lab work, appropriate orders in place, necessary body markings made, patient education given, and so on ("Getting things done" in Table 1.1). This is opposed to the role of the PA leader who has oversight of patient outcomes from surgery, requiring effective preoperative preparations distributed among nurses, technicians, and other APPs routinely carrying out their respective tasks ("Priority consensus" in Table 1.1). While there can be and often is overlap as leaders may be required to manage certain tasks, the APP's role should generally fall on the right side of the column of Table 1.1 if he or she is a leader.

EXPLANATIONS OF LEADERSHIP

Definitions of leadership are more fully explained by descriptions of the leader's attributes or the circumstances surrounding the leader. Four distinct explanations of leadership will be considered throughout this text that better define the role of the leader:

» **Traits:** the personality, motives, values, and skills of the leader

» **Behavior:** the actions, responsibilities, and functions of the leader

» **Power-Influence:** the amount and type of power exercised by the leader

» **Situation:** the nature of the external environment surrounding the leader

Traits

For the APP leader, self-awareness of individual traits is important to recognize, such as if the NP is shy or outgoing, an extrovert or an introvert, a perfectionist or more accepting of failure, and having years of experience or minimal past experience.

Behavior

The actions of the leader are critical as the measure of what produced the outcome, so that achievement of goals is directly related to how the APP led the health care team. To take decisive actions, the responsibilities given to the APP leader must be clear and understood by the health care team. For example, a fallacy of leadership is granting responsibility to a PA without also giving the PA the authority over the area of the responsibility. If the PA is asked to be on-call to make decisions on inpatient sleep hygiene needs for a weekend but the nursing staff is questioning the PA's orders or even unwilling to call the PA, the responsibility given to the PA will not be effective. The functions and responsibilities of the PA must be clear to all members of the health care team.

Power-Influence

Establishing the authority of the APP is then necessary, which institutes various roles for exercising power. For example, the NP may find that certain individuals on the team respond to a more conversational discussion of actions needed compared to other team members who need specific instructions. "Dr. Potter typically wants to be provided a full patient history, an examination report, and a couple options for next steps when a care plan decision is needed," even when the NP knows what is likely the best direction. However, "if Dr. Jones is consulted, she typically expects a short report and a single option for the care plan decision" brings the desired response.

This example of the APP's use of influence portrays the participative leadership role that is instrumental to the APP role. On the surface, there is yet the historical structure of the physician being consulted as the highest position of leadership. However, the NP here has been granted authority and responsibility for a patient's care and, with that, the NP is utilizing powers of influence to bring about the best patient outcomes as identified by the NP leader.

Chapter 2 is dedicated to further exploring power and influence.

Situation

The external factors in the environment of the APP can be the most difficult to control and navigate, and they require individual consideration as much as possible. The PA who works primarily at a family medicine rural satellite clinic open 5 days/week with a physician on-site one-half day each week will have leadership challenges that are different from the PA's challenges who is among four other APPs in a pediatric clinic with eight pediatricians in-house at all times.

NATURE VERSUS NURTURE IN LEADERSHIP

Debate remains over whether leadership is an innate skill that some have and some have not. A review of even recent history suggests that there are those who appear born to be leaders and quickly assume significant and powerful leadership roles primarily by lineage or natural ability. This is especially true when scanning the centuries of time, identifying strong leaders of dynasties, cults, and politics. Engaging stories tell of a seemingly innate talent rising from nowhere with power and influence to direct a large population. Adding further evidence, a genetic link to leadership is suggested in studies of twins that reveal heritable leadership characteristics (Johnson et al., 1998).

However, it is clear that there are teachable leadership skills that are identifiable in more practical situations that likely are common to all. While individuals wielding these skills may not become historical figures of international repute, there is no debate that each person who desires is able to master leadership skills. Those who may have charisma or talents that facilitate their rise to leadership positions will benefit from honing those skills. Those who may not find natural abilities yet still desire to be leaders are not at a disadvantage and with training and practice can become effective.

APPLICATION OF LEADERSHIP RESEARCH METHODOLOGIES

The scientific process, upheld as the primary source of knowledge in medicine, is notably incongruent with the study of leadership. This can become a stumbling block for the APP who seeks best-practice models for determining leadership strategies.

This potential frustration to the clinician seeking to learn about leading stems from the philosophy of Positivism that is fluid throughout science and medicine. This philosophy finds that information derived from sensory experience, logical pathways, and mathematical data are the exclusive source of authoritative knowledge. Though Positivism began to fade in philosophical circles in the mid-20th century, it remains pervasive in Western medicine among those who hold to requiring clear evidence to prove that leadership is effective.

The study of leadership often requires qualitative and mixed methods research to explore the depth of behavioral and social dynamics. While questionnaires, typically based on opinions and perspectives, bring data to the research table, survey results leave much room for interpretation. Clinicians are accustomed to reading about research in a controlled environment with few variables, one of which is controlled by the researcher (the independent variable) to measure the effect of that variable. An example would be using a new drug (the independent variable) for hypertension in a population of individuals carefully screened to be of similar ages, gender, ethnicity, diets, and health. Measuring sequential blood pressures on each individual over months to determine if a specific dose of the drug is effective would typically result in quantitative data to indicate any trends of success or failure. However, trying to similarly control an environment to determine if a particular leadership style yields success is much more difficult. Screening the population by various personalities would be daunting, maintaining a consistent leader influence to each member of the study population would be unwieldy, and determining an outcome of the leadership intervention measured by individual observations would lead to multiple variations in perspective.

That does not mean leadership research should be avoided; in fact, health care systems are gaining much from the exploration of leadership theories and their applications in clinical environments. This text will report on various leadership research outcomes that relate well to clinical settings. While this research is meaningful, the direct application of leadership strategies under study should typically be considered with caution due to the complex situations, other uncontrolled variables, and risk of unintentional effects remaining at play (Spoelstra, Butler, & Delaney, 2016).

SUMMARY POINTS

1. Leadership as it applies to the roles of PAs and NPs is defined as the ability to influence others toward achieving a specific goal.

2. The top-down hierarchical model of leadership based on different levels of authority and power are less common in many team-based organizations including health care. Participative models of leadership that engage common roles of APPs are effective in allowing them to influence others regardless of position or authority.

3. Clinical management is often more task-oriented, involving organizing and carrying out action plans and monitoring results. In contrast, clinical leadership has more to do with casting a vision and explaining innovations or adaptations to new circumstances so that others are motivated to work together in achieving better outcomes.

4. While some people seem to possess natural abilities to lead, every APP has leadership opportunities from individual patient care to working in organizations, using leadership skills that are commonly learned over time. Being intentional in mastering these skills then will bring about more effective leadership.

5. Clinical research is expected to depend on controlling variables to measure outcomes that are commonly clearly defined. Behavioral research about leadership is often less clear as there are many variables that cannot be controlled and the outcomes often are measured by individual perceptions rather than objective measures. However, over time, research outcomes about leadership offer models that suggest

more predictable outcomes. The more this behavioral research is conducted and shared, the clearer the applications will be to represent successful leadership practices.

REFERENCES

Bennis, W. G., & Nanus, B. (1985). *Leaders: The strategies for taking charge.* New York, NY: Harper & Row.

Drucker, P. (1996). The leader of the future. In F. Hesselbein, M. Goldsmith, & R. Beckard (Eds.). *The Peter F. Drucker Foundation for Nonprofit Management.* San Francisco, CA: Jossey-Bass.

Johnson, A. M., Vernon, P. A., McCarthy, J. M., Molson, M., Harris, J. A., & Jang, K. I. (1998). Nature vs nurture: Are leaders born or made? A genetic investigation of leadership style. *Twin Research, 1,* 216–223.

Spoelstra, S., Butler, N., & Delaney, H. (2016). Never let an academic crisis go to waste: Leadership studies in the wake of journal retractions. *Leadership, 12*(4), 383–397.

2

POWER AND INFLUENCE

CRITICAL THINKING QUESTIONS

» **How are advanced practice providers (APPs) able to influence others on the health care team using sources of relational power?**

» **How are patient outcomes improved by the effective use of power?**

» **What methods of influence are more effective in clinical environments when working with different members of the health care team?**

POWER IN THE CONTEXT OF LEADERSHIP

In the leadership definition applied in this book, *the ability to influence others toward achieving a specific goal*, the lead statement is, "the ability to influence others." This identifies the concept of *power*, which holds far-reaching implications within the word. While less attractive words such as "control," "authority," "force," and "domination" can be associated with power, in the context of leadership, power speaks of the capacity to influence others. If one has power, one has the ability to influence. The discussion then turns to how that power should be exercised in achieving a specific goal.

CASE STUDY 1

Pam, a family nurse practitioner (FNP), sees a 55-year-old African American male patient, John, in the evening hours of the adult medicine clinic in central Oregon, 3 hours' drive from a tertiary care hospital. She is a sole provider on this shift and John, who drove himself alone to the clinic, complains of chest pain. Pam knows John from past routine care and he's not a complainer; he typically manages his long-standing diabetes fairly well. Today John describes a central chest pain that is "a heavy weight on my chest" and hasn't relented for 2 hours. He is diaphoretic but denies nausea, and vital signs are stable. His history includes a father and brother who both died in their 60s from myocardial infarctions. Pam obtains a stat ECG that reveals new ST elevations in leads II, III, and AVF, confirming her suspicions. "John, all indications point to this being a myocardial infarction, a heart attack. There's a portion of your heart muscle that is not getting oxygen, likely because of a blockage of your coronary arteries. I've called the emergency unit as we need to have you go right to Central Community Hospital Emergency Room. We'll want to move as fast as we can so we can help open that blockage and save your heart muscle. If we don't act right away, we may have some serious heart problems that are life-threatening."

John interrupts her to say emphatically, "I'm not going to the hospital."

Power is then relational. The ability to influence requires that there be something or someone to influence. Consider the patient in Case Study 1. Pam must now immediately determine how best to influence John to agree to a transfer to receive the care he needs; his life likely depends on it. Pam has the option to use coercion to force him to go, taking the extreme measure of bringing in higher authorities to physically move him, or she can use her relational skills of influence to convince him that her direction must be followed. Before determining next steps in this case study, the full scope of power and influence for the APP should be explored.

THE APP AND POWER

In the world of physician assistants (PAs) and nurse practitioners (NPs), the direction of power may go upward, downward, or laterally because of the many health care team relationships. As well, the APP is on the receiving end of power exercised by others. John offers an example of this bidirectional influence, as he holds power and seeks to influence Pam just as she is trying to persuade him. Recognizing these directions of influence is critical for the APP, as frustration and disruption occur when the power roles are dysfunctional or abusive.

Left to itself, any relationship with a physician, professional peer, supervisor, administrator, or a patient evolves subliminally. If the direction is haphazard, the resulting impact at some point likely touches patient care, raising the stakes for a good outcome. It is the responsibility of the APP to intentionally develop these relationships and use skills of influence to achieve a specific goal and bring about the best outcome.

The traditional hierarchy of the role of the APP in a typical primary care clinic setting may fit the organizational charts shown in Figure 2.1. Either administration or physicians are at the top of the chart, the APP is seen as the next step in the chain of command, then it passes through traditional nursing roles, with allied health services as optional parallel support services when needed. This hierarchy is currently in the flux of change and those clinics using this traditional model are likely becoming fewer, though the mindset is still common.

In actuality, each member of the health care team holds a role with bidirectional influence. Figure 2.2 shows this model for the APP, illustrating that surrounding the APP are health care team members. This holds the opportunity to influence any team member, as well as the opportunity for those team members to influence the APP. If utilized intentionally, skills of influence will then shape the team's ability to achieve the specific goal. For example, consider the lowest relationship in the traditional hierarchy, the role of the clerical staff. If the clinic's appointment scheduler wishes to negatively

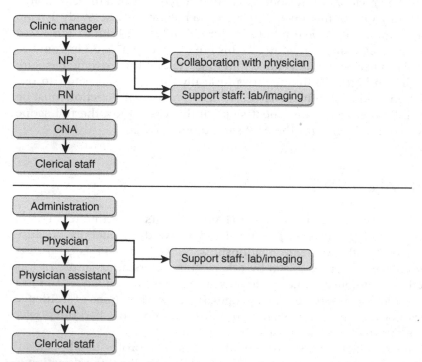

FIGURE 2.1 Outdated hierarchical models of an out-patient clinical organization.

CNA, certified nursing assistant; NP, nurse practitioner; RN, registered nurse.

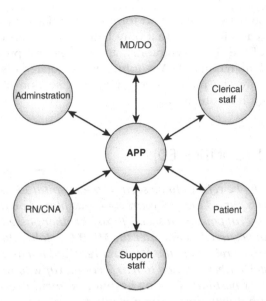

FIGURE 2.2 Advanced practice provider's paths of bidirectional influence.

APP, advanced practice provider; CNA, certified nursing assistant; DO, Doctor of Osteopathic Medicine; RN, registered nurse.

influence the role of the PA, all that is necessary is a tone of voice or subtle comments that would direct a patient to opt out of seeing the PA, perhaps limiting access to care. From the opposite direction, the PA who values the appointment scheduler by affirming the effort given in managing a difficult schedule will likely find a patient schedule that is full and balanced for the PA as controlled by the scheduler, yielding improved access to care.

It is often up to the one who self-identifies as a leader to determine the direction of this influence. If the scheduler exerts a leadership role over the PA, the results often may reflect how much the scheduler likes or dislikes the PA. If the PA exerts a leadership role over the scheduler, the PA likely will control the output of the scheduler by the effectiveness of the PA's leadership skills.

THE PATIENT'S INFLUENCE

The bidirectional influence with the patient is often unrecognized. While by external position the clinician is viewed as having authority and control, the patient may often disagree. As seen in Case Study 1, John wields his power to say whether or not he is going to the hospital. He maintains he has a right to refuse the hospital transport, against the advice of Pam, the NP.

The impasse between Pam and John is potentially life-threatening to John, but in this case, it may be that only Pam understands this because of her knowledge of the signs, symptoms, and the natural progression of an acute myocardial infarction (MI). Yet, John has formulated his own response in refusing the care she recommends. The next section of Case Study 1 further explores John's situation.

CASE STUDY 1 (CONTINUED)

Pam asks John why he refuses to be seen at the hospital ER and learns that John's brother, who passed away 5 years ago, was placed on a blood thinner that he refers to as "rat poison." It seems John's brother passed away due to a cranial bleed that occurred weeks after the MI. While John always associated his brother's death as related to the MI, Pam realized it was probably due to other causes post-MI, likely related to warfarin therapy. John was adamant that the community hospital, the only hospital in town, was responsible for his brother's death due to the treatments given.

Pam seeks to assure John that warfarin ("rat poison") would not be used in his immediate care and could be avoided in the future as other options are available, reiterating that his current chest pain needed immediate treatment. John's response is, "I'd rather die here than in that god-forsaken place."

SOURCES OF POWER

John is exerting a power that is based on what he has learned from his own experience with his brother's demise. This type of "information power" is at odds with Pam's own information power on how to recognize and treat an acute MI. A stalemate is reached as each side is holding to their individual in-formation power. Recognizing this clash of information power offers additional options for Pam, as there are other sources of power from which to draw.

A taxonomy of power sources utilized in leadership research based on the work of French and Raven (1959) addresses five categories of relational power: *legitimate power, coercive power, reward power, referent power,* and *expert power.* Later, a sixth base of power, *information,* was added (Raven, 1965). These remain the classic standard for exploring influence in relationships, often dyadic, where one person seeks to influence the other. More recently, *ecological power* was added as a seventh category of power, initially presented as a form of influence called "situational engineering" (Cartwright, 1965).

Legitimate Power

The formal authority stemming from the position within the organizational hierarchy defines legitimate power. This implies a traditional top-down flow of influence, which is under criticism in application for APPs as the ability to influence upward is recognized (e.g., the NP influencing a physician to achieve a specific goal). In this more authoritarian model, the patient holds an implicit mutual understanding with a clinician that grants the clinician legitimate authority in directing health care decisions. Case Study 1 exhibits ineffective legitimate authority as John does not concede to her recommendation of care.

Coercive Power

If the person influencing another has the ability to institute penalties for not following the leader, the threat of the penalty serves as coercive power. In the workplace, this is represented by an employer threatening to dismiss an employee for not loyally following the leader. This form of power has fallen out of favor out of respect for employee rights. Its application remains real but may unfortunately take subtler forms, often with undertones of unethical or inappropriate use. In health care teams, there may be repercussions of being assigned more time on call or forced to work in less-than-desirable environments as forms of using coercive power. While debate is deserved on applications of coercive power, particularly when used in covert or subversive ways, clear consequences for incompetence or dereliction may be appropriate.

In Case Study 1, Pam's option of using direct coercive power, perhaps tempting in the face of a life-threatening outcome, would not be appropriate. However, it is not uncommon that patients may use the threat of a malpractice accusation as an example of coercive power.

Pam may consider reinforcing the natural consequences of John's inaction, though this is founded primarily in her information against his. If Pam can persuade John that the risk of not following her recommendation of hospital transport is too great, with a potential outcome of a loss of his life, he may concede. From his perspective, it may feel coercive, though it is likely more attributed to Pam's providing clarity in the information at hand, as Pam is unable to control the potential of a negative outcome.

Reward Power

This power is the opposite of coercive power; the person influencing another has the ability to grant rewards to achieve influence. In the business sector, this typically requires that the person has the authority to grant material benefits, which generally occurs in top-down fashion, using pay increases or bonuses as financial incentives. However, reward power can also be applied in exchanging favors, and those lower in the hierarchical order may use reward power as bringing an accolade to or advancing the reputation of the leader.

Between the clinician–patient relationship, reward power is typically intangible. Between Pam and John in Case Study 1, Pam may consider emphasizing how John's life is truly in the balance and how he would gain the reward of a better health outcome by following her recommendation for immediate transport to the hospital. Pam needs to determine if she can be persuasive enough to use reward power in this way, or consider other types of rewards (e.g., what family members may want that John would see as a benefit). While Pam may not have authority over granting those rewards, using the benefits of a positive outcome, particularly if John is cognizant of the high risk of this as a life or death decision, may convince him to go to the hospital.

Ecological Power

Control over the organization's structure, such as work environments and technology, brings this newer source of power. The utilization of electronic medical records (EMRs) may either advance or hinder, thereby influencing, the outcome. Those able to control the function of EMR are able to directly guide the effectiveness of the health care environment, both in the quality of care and in job satisfaction.

Those who develop the organizational structure of health care delivery systems also influence the related outcomes. Whether it be health care administrators running a hospital, governmental agencies establishing health care policies, or the individual APP exploring the path to a consultant needed for a patient referral, this source of ecological power has clear implications. For Case Study 1, the fact that there is only one hospital in the community limits the application of ecological power in the medical care decisions necessary for John.

Information Power

Examples of information power as applied in Case Study 1 have been described earlier in this chapter, illustrating how possession of information and controlling its release can be strongly influential.

In the varying relationships among the health care team, each party holds different aspects of information. Consider the following examples of information available from these members of a health care team:

» The pharmacist may have information related to drug side effects.

» The social worker may have information about a patient's ability to pay.

» The physical therapist will have information on the compliance of a patient receiving treatments.

» The nutritionist will have information related to the patient's dietary practice.

» The hospital nurse will have information on how the patient fared overnight.

These team members all have control over their respective reports and determine what to share, hopefully in an environment that allows the free exchange of vital information. There are situations where the disclosure of information may be deleterious, such as when the APP or physician has information regarding limited institutional resources. Divulging these concerns may be withheld if such information shared with the team would disrupt an individual patient's outcomes.

POSITION POWERS AND PERSONAL POWERS

The sources of power described up to this point (legitimate, coercive, reward, ecological, and information) are powers of position. In a relationship between two individuals or within a group, these sources of power are inherent to the position held by the leader. Legitimate power is directly linked to the authority granted to the person in that position. If one has the ability to administer penalties, he or she has coercive power, and similarly, if the person is able to distribute resources or offer benefits, reward power is exercised. If the position holds the privilege of information that is not accessible by another, information power is at play. Figure 2.3 displays these five position powers with varying degrees of influence for the leader. Central in the figure are the two forms of personal power.

Expert and referent power are examples of a personal power. These either come from attributes of the individual or arise from the personal aspects of the relationship. Friendship and loyalty influence personal power, as the source of power does not come from position but from the talents or personality of the individual or the social dynamic of the relationship.

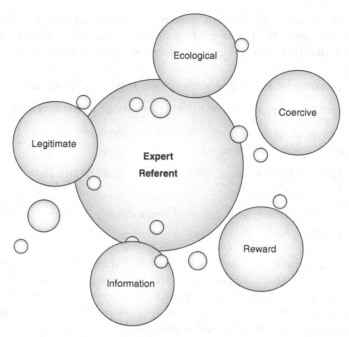

FIGURE 2.3 Personal powers in relationship with position powers.

Expert Power

The challenge of expert power is that the one to be influenced must respect that the person who seeks to influence others truly has expertise. As this expertise comes from both knowledge and experience, there is overlap between the use of information power and expert power. A person with a wealth of wisdom and skill mastery exercises expert power as long as others are dependent on needing this expertise and recognizing who possesses it.

In health care, this is a personal power because the individual must be reliable in providing information and trusted in leading well to have the influence of expert power that will yield results. Once the level of expertise is no longer needed, others are no longer dependent on those with this power. Misuse of expert power occurs if the individual seeks to keep his or her expertise as a secret or avoids teaching others the knowledge and skills, serving only to maintain possession of expert power.

It has been suggested that in patient-centered health care, the patients should be given the knowledge needed to make their own decisions, which challenges the notion of expert power. It makes the assumption that this expert power, by way of transference of knowledge, can be given to the patient. The patient then would hold the ultimate responsibility for his or her own health care decisions. However, the level of expertise required typically is far more complex than what can be conveyed in a clinician–patient relationship (Canter, 2001).

Expert power has already failed in Case Study 1 since John does not respect that Pam holds expertise. Pam's credentials may be misunderstood. She could seek to give evidence of her expertise in an effort to persuade John that she can be trusted, but it is a time-consuming risk that may not yield a benefit.

Referent Power

Referent power is recognized completely at the discretion of those being influenced. It refers to having the respect and esteem of others so that they wish to support the goals and carry out the requests of the leader. Strong referent power exists between friends or with someone who is the recipient of great affection or admiration, often stemming from the person's character traits of integrity and compassion. Dynamic and beloved individuals often possess referent power, leading some to call this "charismatic power." It may seem to hold an almost supernatural command, perhaps founded in misplaced adulation. Some administrators, physicians, APPs, or other leaders have such a strong charismatic personality that they find environments where they can lead decision making easily without debate. On the other hand, an authentic leader who upholds virtues without reproach may have earned referent power and may be able to use that power for the benefit of all.

In Case Study 1, Pam should reassess how John responds to her to determine if she possesses even a small amount of referent power on which to depend. If John would recognize her as a person of integrity who sincerely seeks the best for him, he may respond with reluctant acceptance to her recommendations.

All seven sources of power offer opportunities for impact depending on the relationship and situation. While the aforementioned descriptions are directed toward the clinician/patient relationship illustrated in Case Study 1, these sources of influence apply among all relationships in the health care team. Table 2.1 offers further guidelines for the APP using each power when appropriate in a health care situation.

TABLE 2.1 Guidelines for Using Sources of Power in Health Care Teams

Power	Guidelines
Legitimate	Firm, confident leadership is expected without apology Actions should be clearly understood by others The boundaries of authority should be established and not exceeded
Coercive	Warnings and penalties should be dealt personally and confidentially Consequences should be implemented promptly without favoritism Actions should maintain the intent of helping to reach the goal
Reward	Rewards should equal what was promised Avoid use of rewards to invite competition within the team
Information	Openly clarify information without political spin Admit when additional information is needed and obtain it Avoid information dumping, excessively sharing more details than necessary
Ecological	Adapt systems and structures to the team, rather than making the team adapt to the system or structure Assure physical work environments are conducive to best practice (adequate lighting, equipment, temperature, flow of traffic, etc.)
Expert	Be decisive with clear reasoning Avoid exaggeration and misinformation Support actions by building on past success when possible
Referent	Visibly demonstrate personal commitment Be genuine in appreciating affirmation Participate in the actions needed Share in any required sacrificial time or effort

CASE STUDY 1 (CONTINUED)

Pam, standing in the clinic room as John sat stewing over their debate, recognized that this clash of information was not effective. At this point, she needs to use her influence from a different source. She lowers her voice and appeals to him with referent power.

"John, I want you to know that my commitment is to provide the best care that I can for you. I've always dealt straight with you; I don't believe you'll find that I've ever led you the wrong way. I know you're understandably scared right now, and you need to be able to trust that we are here to do all we can to help you."

John is silent but seems less belligerent. Pam continues, taking a chair to sit across from him, accessing her source of expert power. "I've seen too many individuals with your symptoms and while we're never 100% sure, your symptoms are classic for a heart attack. I think you know it's serious because of how you feel. Right now, you need someone you can trust, and I am convinced based on my clinical experience and knowledge of your condition that this is the right direction."

She then adds an exchange of favors, representing reward power. "I'm very comfortable in my recommendation to you, and I know the emergency room staff that will be caring for you. If you will go now, I will speak directly with them to make sure they are aware of your situation and your concerns over your brother's unfortunate experience. And I will be able to come see you shortly at the hospital to be sure you are finding the care you expect.

"The emergency unit should be here any minute. I'll call your family. Can we help you get ready?"

There are APPs who have a natural affinity for using sources of power, and you, the reader, may find intuitively that you have your own approach and language to address John and his situation. The emphasis here is intentionally noting the use of sources of power, when one source of power may be more effective than another, and how they offer an additive effect when combined. Learning by trial-and-error which sources of power are most effective for the individual APP provides an array of resources in guiding patient management and best outcomes. The APP who understands and intentionally operates sources of power will undoubtedly find more career success and better patient outcomes.

INFLUENCE TACTICS ON THE HEALTH CARE TEAM

On the health care team, the sources of power are bidirectionally active as described earlier in this chapter. Often this influence occurs spontaneously if not reactively when a health care team is asked to take on a new responsibility. Tasks that come before health care teams are opportunities for the APP to offer leadership, such as the following examples:

» Developing a more streamlined process to deliver critical care consultation reports to the primary care provider

» Creating an evaluation process to measure patient outcomes in a specific department

» Revising a clinical staffing system that adequately covers evening and weekend hours of health services without overly taxing the providers

These and many other worthwhile projects that advance productive health care delivery require the APP to be skilled and in position to influence the team toward the goal of improved health care outcomes.

The sources of power presented up to this point in this chapter are the toolboxes that leaders use. Inside the box are influence tactics that serve as the actual hammers and wrenches the leader would need. In the hands of a skilled leader, these influence tactics are actions proactively performed by the leader to guide others toward the desirable goal. APPs will find that these influence tactics, used in the context of a hierarchical leadership, may be directed upward to superiors, lateral to peers, or downward to those being led by the APP. As health care teams continue to evolve without such organized hierarchy, these tactics may offer the APP a variety of options in influencing others to achieve a goal.

Research in the business and management fields since the 1980s has explored tactics surrounding critical incidents that required the direct influence of the leader, and measures have been applied to determine what leads to a successful and unsuccessful influence attempt. The research is not nearly as robust in exploring these attempts in the health care arena, but there are lessons to learn. Yukl and his colleagues (2013) have conducted a series of studies over the past two decades and described 11 influence tactics used by leaders in management settings, determining that four are generally of high effectiveness, four are moderately effective, and three tend toward low effectiveness (Table 2.2). The impact of each influence tactic is highly dependent on the individual situation and the leader's effectiveness in using the tactic. Understanding this taxonomy of influence tactics will provide the tools that may be effective within different sources of power, leader applications, and health care settings. The grouping of these tactics here will guide the leader to appreciate the benefits and risks of their applications.

TABLE 2.2 Influence Tactics Based on Effectiveness*

High Effectiveness	Moderate Effectiveness	Low Effectiveness
Rational Persuasion**	Apprising	Coalition tactic
Inspirational Appeal	Ingratiation	Legitimating tactic
Consultation**	Exchange	Pressure
Collaboration	Personal appeal	

*Effectiveness categorization adapted from Yukl (2013, p. 207).
**Effectiveness additionally supported by Sampson (2012, pp. 46–48).

Influence Tactics of High Effectiveness

RATIONAL PERSUASION

This proactive tactic involves giving clear evidence and logical support to achieve an important task. If the team does not already have unity toward working together for a desired outcome, this tactic may not be effective. The leader should also have sufficient background, if not expertise, in the project's substance. However, if a team is functioning well, a knowledgeable leader's appeal that involves factual evidence with thoughtfully predicted outcomes offers a proactive step that will yield a greater potential of success.

INSPIRATIONAL APPEAL

As opposed to the logical arguments presented earlier in rational persuasion, this proactive tactic seeks to appeal to the team in finding value in achieving a goal. By defining how the team's hopes and ideals will be met, this tactic may best be applied when seeking a commitment to working on a new project, or addressing a significant change from past methods.

CONSULTATION

Consultation as a tactic is distinct from the clinical reference of a patient consultation. As a proactive influence tactic, consultation refers to the leader inviting selected team members into the planning of a project. With this, the project's objective is not under consideration but is predetermined. The consultation is devoted to how the objective should be achieved. Those selected for consultation by the leader should already be supportive of the project, so that the tactic will further explore issues of feasibility and potential obstacles.

COLLABORATION

This last of the four influence tactics that have shown high effectiveness is the leader clearly communicating to the team that all resources and assistance will be available for the project. This provides assurance to the team that attention has been given to reduce potential difficulties related to inadequate resources. This tactic is at times neglected, as the team would assume that all support needed for a project will be provided. The use of this influence tactic by the leader intentionally addresses this available support so that the team can place more confidence in its own success. This influence tactic is less effective if there is a question of reliability or history of inadequate resources in support of past projects.

All of these four influence tactics were found to be of high effectiveness in the studies of management settings by Yukl and colleagues. Additionally, two of these tactics, rational persuasion and consultation, were also found to be effective in a separate study of physicians and allied health providers at a large Australian health organization (Sampson, 2012).

Influence Tactics of Moderate Effectiveness

APPRISING
The influence tactic of apprising by the leader is communicating that there is a clear benefit to the individual or team conducting the proposed project. The success of the project would advance the goals of the organization, but this tactic clarifies the more personal benefit that the team will gain.

INGRATIATION
When sincere, the leader's actions in being abundantly helpful if not friendly to the team is an influence tactic that has intended results of the team further appreciating and valuing the leader. Genuine praise and compliments coming from the leader can be powerful as a proactive influence tactic. When it occurs in the context of then immediately asking for something in return, it will be interpreted as manipulative and likely be damaging to the team.

EXCHANGE
The use of the exchange tactic can be a liability, as it promises a reward to the team for doing what is asked. If the project has no other benefits of value, this may be necessary, but otherwise it likely serves little to advance health care delivery. The liability behind this tactic is that the promised benefit typically is a monetary compensation or other tangible incentive that must be delivered. If there are mixed interpretations of what is required to participate in the project, attempting to withhold the reward because the leader is not satisfied by the team's performance will likely lead to discord.

PERSONAL APPEAL
Using personal appeals is akin to asking for personal favors. It may be more effective to use a personal appeal laterally to a peer outside of the team, as opposed to upward or downward within the team. Offering a personal appeal upward to a superior by the APP may be confused as favoritism. Downward or otherwise within a team of peers, asking for a favor risks offense as it comes across as pleading or unfairly placing a burden on the team.

Influence Tactics of Low Effectiveness

COALITION TACTIC
This tactic identifies others outside the team to add their endorsement if not influence to the team's efforts. It often occurs only because the team itself either is inadequate for the task or is unwilling to proceed. Yukl and

colleagues classified coalition tactics between moderate and low effectiveness, perhaps as it may be more effective in situations where the appeal goes upward, to convince superiors of a direction of a project.

LEGITIMATING TACTIC

Legitimating tactic is used primarily when the team is not familiar with the leader's credibility or expertise. If legitimacy is questioned, relationships among the team are likely indistinct, suggesting that there may be multiple obstacles within the group dynamic that may require attention.

PRESSURE

Pressure tactics involve the leader making repeated inquiries of progress, perhaps even with warnings or threats to provoke desired action or behavior from the team. While it may lead to accomplishing the tasks at hand, it also creates a defensive atmosphere within the team, leading to resentful attitudes.

Those influence tactics marked by low effectiveness should not necessarily be avoided, but caution is necessary, as is true for those categorized as moderately effective. Those labeled at high effectiveness offer no guarantee of success but have more of a track record of acceptance and desired results. Case Study 2 offers a scenario to explore the utilization of these influence tactics by an APP.

CASE STUDY 2

Mark is the senior PA on a team of five APPs and five surgeons, plus nursing and ancillary staff support in a busy orthopedic practice. He has been called to meet with the department director and Dr. Garza, the lead surgeon for the knee team. The department has a contract to utilize a new laparoscopic device that leads to shorter hospital stays and better outcomes in multiple published studies. Use of the device will require on-site training for all members of the surgical team, scheduled for a 4-week period with the medical device company, 3 months from now. The director and Dr. Garza are asking Mark to lead the implementation of this new device with appropriate training. Expectations include a minimum of five procedures completed with the new device by each surgeon and measured outcomes of provider satisfaction, OR time, hospital length-of-stay, patient outcomes, and patient satisfaction.

Mark is aware that the team is already consumed with the high volume of procedures from the past 6 months, and morale among the PAs has been tenuous at times, though they are compensated well for their work, including a lucrative over-time pay differential. The physicians on the team are all highly respected. Each APP seems to enjoy the work relationships, if it were not for the long hours including the frequent additional shifts, which are typically shared by all.

The director asks that there be a minimal reduction of surgical case volume. The expectation that the device brings shorter hospital stays should allow increased procedures compared to the current pace to offset the training time needed in the early course of the implementation process. Dr. Garza adds that he will see that additional support staff is in place, loaned temporarily from the hand team due to one of its surgeons being on maternity leave.

Mark agrees to bring this to the team of APPs and develop a plan for the implementation process with the required evaluation measures.

What proactive influence tactics may be most effective for Mark to use, both in achieving the needed support from Dr. Garza and the department director, and from his APP peers?

(Case Study 2 is a student exercise to explore the strategy and application of influence tactics. If the reader has real-life work situations that can be explored by considering what influence tactics may be effective to use, this likely enriches the exercise.)

SUMMARY POINTS

1. APPs are expected to have strong relationships in their professional roles with all members of the health care team, spanning the spectrum of those with higher and lower authority. Even in a more traditional hierarchy of structure, APPs are centrally positioned to interact almost equally upward and downward in the order. This fosters strong peer relationships in the health care setting. It also conveys a more lateral relationship at times with patients compared to the typical doctor–patient relationship, which not only brings the strength of open communication but also may create obstacles if the APP's position of authority is not respected.

2. Sources of power, when effectively applied, allow health care teams to function efficiently in reaching goals. If appropriate goals are pursued, patient outcomes are likely to improve. The two personal power sources of referent and expert powers are at the disposal of all APPs. The position powers of legitimate, coercive, reward, information, and ecological powers are associated directly with the responsibilities and authority of the individual APP in the specific medical setting. The haphazard use of sources of power can yield unpredictable results, and the power of influence in professional relationships may be misused. However, the APP who understands these seven sources of power will

intentionally utilize skills of influence, respectful of all team members. Such leadership effectively supports the attainment of the goals of the team, which are often focused on improved patient outcomes.

3. The APP is uniquely positioned to influence the health care team as a leader, with impact both upward to superiors of the team and lateral and downward to other team members. With a variety of different influence tactics from which to draw, those that seem most effective in many management settings include rational persuasion, inspirational appeal, consultation, and collaboration. When the APP has an opportunity to lead proactively, consideration of these influence tactics may be predictive of success. A number of other influence tactics are identified with less predictive value of success, but may still have application in the particular setting and leadership style of the APP.

REFERENCES

Canter, R. (2001). Patients and medical power (editorial). *British Medical Journal, 323,* 414. doi:10.1136/bmj.323.7310.414

Cartwright, D. (1965). Influence, leadership, and control. In J. G. March (Ed.), *Handbook of organizations* (pp. 1–47). Chicago, IL: Rand McNally.

French, J., & Raven, B. H. (1959). The bases of social power. In D. Cartwright (Ed.), *Studies of social power* (pp. 150–167). Ann Arbor, MI: Institute for Social Research.

Raven, B. H. (1965). Social influences and power. In I. D. Steiner & M. Fishbein (Eds.), *Current studies in social psychology* (pp. 371–381). New York, NY: Holt, Reinhart & Winston.

Sampson, S. (2012). *Influence tactics and leader effectiveness: How effective, contemporary leaders influence subordinates* (Unpublished master's thesis). Queensland University of Technology, Brisbane, Queensland, Australia, pp. 46–48.

Yukl, G. (2013). *Leadership in organizations* (8th ed., pp. 188–215). Upper Saddle River, NJ: Pearson.

3

CLINICAL LEADERSHIP TRAITS

CRITICAL THINKING QUESTIONS

» **Should an advanced practice provider (APP) find a particular personality approach to become a more popular type of leader?**

» **If leadership is unique for different situations, how does an APP discover personal leadership traits that function in a variety of settings?**

» **Is being a charismatic APP preferable for providing the best care for patients and effectively leading health care teams?**

» **How does the APP maintain composure to effectively influence health care system challenges in a high-stress environment?**

PERSONALITY CLASSIFICATION

The personality of a leader brings certain traits that are effective with different types of teams. These traits are distinctive characteristics that are integral to the very nature of the leader. Often, leaders have possessed these traits since birth, seen as innate temperaments, birth order characteristics, or other personality traits. How the APP acts in seeking to influence others will determine his or her success, and those actions will reflect the leader's personality.

In considering personality traits, the "Big Five Personality Factors" are often used to classify an individual's personality, defined in the following (Goldberg, 1990, with original descriptive terms in parentheses):

- **Neuroticism (Affect):** The tendency to be anxious, insecure, timid, and immature, as opposed to being emotionally stable (A "low neuroticism" rating is desirable.)

- **Extraversion (Power):** The tendency to be socially engaged, spirited, and adventuresome

- **Openness (Intellect):** The tendency to be insightful, original, and knowledgeable

- **Agreeableness (Love):** The tendency to be accepting, trusting, tolerant, and generous

- **Conscientiousness (Work):** The tendency to be organized, industrious, dependable, and disciplined

Researchers have attempted to identify relationships among these five personality types and leadership, though most studies of this type are completed primarily in business and management fields. In an oft-cited article, Judge, Bono, Ilies, and Gerhardt (2002) conducted a meta-analysis of 78 leadership studies published between 1967 and 1998, finding that extraversion, conscientiousness, openness, and low neuroticism were associated with leadership; agreeableness was only weakly associated. However, in some specific styles of leadership, the findings are different. In a study of 14 samples of leadership across 200 organizations, extraversion, agreeableness, and openness were associated with the transformational style of leadership; conscientiousness and neuroticism were unrelated to this leadership style (Judge & Bono, 2000). As these two studies show, extraversion is a common personality type associated with effective leadership (see later in this chapter in the context of a charismatic leader). The other four personality types are less clearly associated with leadership. These studies do not focus on health care team models, so the leadership correlation with personality types may be even less apparent.

While the classification of personality related to leadership may be difficult, the APP must be aware of his or her personality related to how leadership skills are applied. While completely changing a personality is not possible or expected, the APP's personality can be self-adjusted according to what is needed to influence the team.

In addition to being self-aware of his or her own personality, considering the individual personalities of the team members helps the APP effectively influence the group. The team member who is clearly conscientious, as categorized by the Big Five, will function well if the team is organized and has clear goals planned. The team member whose personality leans toward agreeableness is counted on when support is needed. The team member who tends toward neuroticism will need emotional support. The individual who reflects openness will bring new ideas. The one who shows extraversion will bring enthusiasm and energy toward the success of the team.

A SITUATIONAL APPROACH TO LEADING

A common approach to leadership gives attention to the specific gathering of individuals being led. As the APP focuses on influencing others on the team, the abilities and personalities of the team members are important to understand to determine what skills of influence are needed. If the APP finds that there are arrogant or disinterested personalities on the team, this requires a different approach; so too, the team that has individuals with little experience compared to team members that have years of experience. The APP then tailors the leadership approach based on the situation represented by the collection of team members.

The individual qualities of each team member make each team different and are constantly changing over time. The external environment and practical resources supporting the team goals are also in a frequent state of flux. The priority of the APP should be in assessing how best to respond to the varying qualities of the team members, which may suggest a specific approach based on the attitudes and skills of all parties involved.

One widely recognized model of this situational approach to leadership is Situational Leadership®, first developed by Hersey, Blanchard, and Johnson (2012), with a range of published studies since the 1970s exploring its use in various organizations. As it is a popular leadership training model, it is commonly found as a model used in health care organizations.

This leadership style divides leadership traits into two patterns, *directive traits* and *supportive traits*. Directive traits guide members by giving specific directions, establishing clear goals, and using timelines, typically in one-direction communication from the leader to the team. Supportive traits are more nurturing by two-way communication using praise, exchanging ideas in problem solving, and offering emotional support. Using a bimodal combination of these two types of traits (a mix of high- and low-degree combinations), a two-by-two diagram establishes four styles of leadership (See Table 3.1). Likely, the APP's personality lends itself to one of the four categories, though in Situational Leadership the leader is expected to adjust to the category of leadership style warranted by the team.

TABLE 3.1 Directive and Supportive Situational Traits in Leadership

Trait	High Directive Trait	Low Directive Trait
High Supportive Trait	High Directive–High Supportive (S2)	Low Directive–High Supportive (S3)
Low Supportive Trait	High Directive–Low Supportive (S1)	Low Directive–Low Supportive (S4)

Directing Style (S1): This is *high directive–low supportive trait*, primarily focused on the leader clearly communicating the directions for achieving the goal, without as much attention to supporting the emotional needs of the team.

Coaching Style (S2): This is a *high directive–high supportive trait*, providing details on how to achieve the goal and nurturing the team by gaining input and providing feedback as the work continues.

Supporting Style (S3): This is a *low directive–high supportive trait* for a team that manages tasks well but needs reinforcement, praise, and an exchange of ideas to make progress.

Delegating Style (S4): This is a *low directive–low supportive trait*, reflecting a team that is self-directed and self-supporting so that the leader can step back and delegate responsibilities to the team.

Situational Leadership in Health Care Teams

A study from the Netherlands explored these situational leadership traits from the perspective of physician supervisors and residents as team members (van der Wal, Scheele, Schönrock-Adema, Jaarsma, & Cohen-Schotanus, 2015). This study is explored as a model of assessing a clinical institution to assess effective leadership.

A dual questionnaire measured situational leadership traits perceived by the physician supervisors themselves and as perceived by the residents. Similar to the aforementioned definitions of situational leadership traits, directive traits of the leader were measured by the degree of specific directions given (exact instructions, high directive) or global directions given (generalized instructions, low directive). Supportive traits of the leader were measured by the degree that the supervisor made mutual decisions with the resident (high supportive), or the supervisor gave a directive and responded to the resident only to clarify instructions (two-way communication, low supportive). In this study, the residents ($N = 117$) reported observing global directions most frequently in the supervisor physicians (86%) and two-way communication next most frequently (73%). Specific instructions (64%) and mutual decision making (59%) were observed less frequently. This would suggest a low directive–low supportive situational leadership trait.

Measuring the self-report of these leadership traits among the supervisor physicians ($N = 201$) revealed similar results. The physicians reported displaying the same two most common traits in themselves, giving global directions (96%) and using two-way communication (91%). Giving specific instruction (57%) and mutual decision making (80%) were displayed less, reversed in order of frequency from the residents scoring (see Table 3.2). So, again, this identifies a low directive–low supportive situational leadership trait.

The authors found that this pattern of a low directive–low supportive leadership trait was consistent at the starting level of the residency, the immediate level, and during the most experienced level of the residency (van der Wal et al., 2015). In situational leadership, leaders should begin with more directive leadership and then advance to more supportive leadership traits as the team members become more experienced, as this is correlated with higher performance and well-being among the team members. In this study, there was no adjustment of leadership over the course of the residency.

Perhaps most telling, the authors noted that one-third of residents reported not observing the traits of being given specific instructions (high directive) or participating in mutual decision making (high supportive) at all as residents (van der Wal et al., 2015). The physician supervisors reported the same with one-third not displaying these traits. The authors conclude that one cannot assume that leadership traits will be appropriately modeled to maximize the residents' performance and well-being, and recommend that physician supervisors need to be taught effective leadership strategies. They also admit that the absence of perceiving or reporting high directive or high supportive leadership traits is because situational leadership is not an appropriate model of leadership in the environment of the study.

TABLE 3.2 Physician Supervisor and Residents Report of Situational Leadership Traits

	Physician Supervisor's Self-Report (N = 201)	Resident's Perceptions of Leader (N = 117)
Directive Leadership		
Global Instructions (Low)	96%	86%
Specific Instructions (High)	57%	64%
Supportive Leadership		
Two-Way Communication (Low)	91%	73%
Mutual Decision Making (High)	80%	59%

Source: van der Wal et al. (2015).

This study is limited as it was conducted at one institution in the Netherlands, so generalizing these results to other environments is not advised. However, it offers a model of exploring the clinical environment to determine leadership effectiveness. Discovering which leadership traits are utilized and if they are adjusted to the team members' competence provides compelling evidence of the potential need for leadership training at the institution.

Team Members in Development

The Situational Leadership II® model (Blanchard, Zigarmi, & Zigarmi, 2013) maintains that the competency and commitment of the team members responding to the leadership style are important to the success of the team. The attributes of the individual team members then become important factors in the leader's ability to influence them toward the goal. This model categorizes the team members across the continuum from "developing" (D1) to "developed" (D4), according to two attributes of the members: commitment (personally striving to achieve the goals) and competence (the skills to effectively perform).

D1 individuals are low in competence but high in commitment, so they are new to the tasks but enthusiastic about the team. D2 individuals are minimally competent and low on commitment, so they lack motivation though likely are capable. D3 individuals have high competence, but variable commitment, so they are capable but it is not clear the job will get done without encouragement. D4 individuals are most favorable with high competence and high commitment, so they are highly motivated and can be expected to perform well.

This gradient of development of the team members is not bimodal like the four categories of leadership. The authors of the model find that most team members are initially eager to learn (D1), then go through a phase of discouragement or disillusionment (D2), leading to a stage of lacking confidence (D3) before returning to full motivation (D4). While somewhat sequential, the lower commitment in stages D2 and D3 seems arbitrary, which is among the criticisms of Situational Leadership II (Northouse, 2016).

SITUATIONAL APPROACH TO LEADERSHIP FOR APPs

Using the Situational Leadership II model, the APP would determine the situation of the team regarding the mix of competence and commitment across the members. The developmental level (D1–D4) is then paired with the same leadership style (S1 with D1, etc.).

Consider the application of this leadership model in a critical care team at a tertiary care hospital.

CASE STUDY 1

Annette is an experienced nurse practitioner (NP) who works three 12-hour shifts/week, mostly nights, in critical care at State University Hospital. Physicians on the team include the chief resident, the attending physician, and the intensivist fellow. Other members include one of the hospital pharmacists, a newly hired social worker, the nutritionist, the current shift's respiratory therapist, critical care nurse, and a couple of health professions students. Together on morning rounds, the team heads in to see Mr. Hart, who has had a rough night under Annette's watch on his third postop day after a multivessel coronary artery bypass graft (CABG).

The intensivist fellow, who has been up through the night with Annette, gives the report, addressing the complicated details of Mr. Hart's condition. The physicians on the team engage in the discussion, asking the pharmacist a number of drug-related questions. Annette listens to the conversation. She knows from an earlier conversation this morning that the nutritionist, Mary, has some suggestions to revise Mr. Hart's dietary support. Mary is shrinking back as the chief resident is making his point to the others. Their conversation reaches a resolution that Annette finds helpful. The attending physician asks the group, "Does that cover what we need here?" as the other two physicians quickly turn and are nearly out the door with the team following their lead.

That's when Annette says, "Mary has a good idea for adjusting the TPN." The attending physician looks at Mary and responds, "Hold up, everyone. Yes, let's look at that."

Among the critical care team, there is always a mix of personalities and traits that must blend to work well. It is important that someone on the team recognize the development of the members, as Annette did in Case Study 1. The Situational Leadership II provides a matrix to help indicate that Mary, the nutritionist, is likely at D2, low to some degree of competence and low commitment. This indicates a need for the S2 style of leadership (paired with D2), which is the high directive–high supportive (coaching) style. So, Annette involves herself by making a simple request that supports Mary and also directs her to give her expert advice (*"Mary has a good idea for adjusting the TPN."*). Annette's actions come from her measure of Mary's development level, having taken the time to listen to the nutritionist earlier that morning. Annette, getting prior input from the team members, being clear in the steps needed to reach the goal, and providing encouragement, demonstrates the S2 style of coaching.

To take the leadership action demonstrated by Annette, a personality change is not necessary. It may be easier for the extraversion personality to speak out during the morning rounds as the team was heading out the door, but the APP with a knowledge of this situational approach to leadership can self-adjust to make this important contribution to the team.

Case Study 1 illustrates the APP in a position of influence laterally or downward. As the APP typically is positioned to have influence upward as well, the next case study gives an example of using the situational approach to leadership in that direction.

CASE STUDY 2

Rachel is a physician assistant (PA) for a general pediatrics clinic of six pediatricians, four other APPs, and sufficient nursing, allied health, and support staff for the busy practice. She has asked to meet with the medical staff leadership at their monthly meeting to share her proposal to implement a weekly asthma clinic. The clinic has explored this in the past and, while the need for consistent asthma management is needed, the patient volume has been in question to support a half-day clinic. Rachel has earlier spoken with three pediatricians and gained their support. Two others seem ambivalent as their respective patient populations are focused on neonatal and behavioral health, and they wish her well with no commitment. One of the other physician owners, Dr. Brown, is likely to be resistant (again) as he believes the patients seen by this asthma clinic will draw down his patient volume. He also questions if the care will meet his expectations. Rachel respects Dr. Brown and acknowledges that he has significant influence over the clinical administrator, Ms. Green, who remains focused on the financial cost/revenue. She legitimately maintains that the asthma clinic will pull a PA from seeing acutely ill walk-in patients. As the acute walk-in patient traffic is a greater volume of revenue than the asthma clinic, which focuses on preventive care for patients with asthma, she predicts this will bring reduced revenue. These two individuals have strong personalities that often sway the decisions of the leadership.

Rachel comes to the meeting with best-practice evidence supporting the clinical design. She has collected data that shows a 2-year, high rate of treatment of patients with acute asthma needs in their clinic. She plans to demonstrate how the asthma clinic would likely improve these patients' asthma management. She has budget projections that give reasonable targets to breakeven in expense/revenue by 6 months. Her fellow APPs support her, though due to the busy patient volume they don't believe they would be asked to participate in the asthma clinic, and their interest is not that high.

Rachel next considers a situational approach to this meeting with the medical leadership. She considers her own personality to be most consistent with "agreeableness" from the Big Five categories. Dr. Brown and Ms. Green are both likely "conscientiousness." She then considers the development levels of her audience and recognizes all are highly competent, but Dr. Brown and Ms. Green are likely on the variable commitment scale for this proposal. That places them both at D3, so her leadership style would need to be S3, the low directive–high supportive (supporting) style. Interpreting this upward to these superiors, she plans to present her objective information, but will avoid a strong emphasis on the evidence and data she has collected (less directive). Her strategy is then to approach the presentation prepared to listen, ask for input, and give feedback, respecting the expertise of the medical leadership (more supportive). Rachel best identifies with the "agreeableness" personality type. This strategy follows the S3 leadership style, helping her adjust to what may be her most effective approach to the leadership in achieving the goal of this asthma clinic.

In Case Study 2, Rachel is equipped with all that she needs to make an effective appeal to her clinical leadership. However, she may wish she was more aligned with the "extraversion" personality type in this presentation. The appeal of the extraversion personality type captivates many who explore what it takes to be a good leader. This personality is most aligned with a leadership style called "charismatic leadership."

THE LEADERSHIP TRAIT OF CHARISMA

Charismata comes from a Greek term referring to "a divinely conferred power or talent" in the Oxford English Dictionary. In leadership, it has been identified as a personality trait that includes the other's perception of the leader's possession of exceptional if not superhuman powers (Weber, 1947). Over time, further leadership research has combined Weber's ideas with a recognition of a more tempered sense of charismatic powers that speak of the confident leader who is able to captivate those around her or him.

Historical figures often identified as charismatic leaders include Napoleon Bonaparte, Winston Churchill, Eva Peron, John F. Kennedy, Fidel Castro, and Nelson Mandela. These figures all demonstrate attributes classically associated with charismatic leadership (Conger & Kanungo, 1998):

» A dynamic vision that is articulated clearly

» An appeal to high morals and shared values

» Pursuing an ideal via unconventional behavior

» Conveying confidence and optimism in the midst of self-sacrifice

Two Theories of Charismatic Leadership in Medicine

It is difficult to find a historical figure in medicine with the broad appeal that represents these characteristics. It may be that charismatic leadership does not fit health care leadership as well as in other leadership opportunities. However, on a more local level, likely there are clinicians who have a popularity among patients and coworkers that seems to surpass what would be expected in view of their otherwise regular skills or temperament. This indicates an important aspect of charismatic leadership: people around the leader determine if the leader exhibits charisma. Called "the attribution theory of charismatic leadership" (Conger & Kanungo, 1998), this proposes that the ability of the individual to lead is based on the perceptions of those following the leader.

Often, the charismatic leader arises from a crisis where the people are fearful or anxious over economic demise, physical danger, or the destruction of values (e.g., leaders who rose in the aftermath of the 9/11 attacks in the United States). In medicine, this is not an uncommon occurrence, as when a patient and family face a major health concern and the clinician is positioned to provide relief and care. The discerning APP needs to recognize the potential of patients attributing exceptional power (charisma) to herself or himself to avoid misusing this perception. The patient or family may believe that the clinician possesses some unusual level of greatness that is not deserved and this should be extinguished to avoid later confusion or impossible expectations.

A different theory exploring charismatic leadership may contribute to improved patient health. The self-concept theory of charismatic leadership (House, 1977; Shamir, House, & Arthur, 1993) finds that charismatic leadership is represented by how those around the leader see themselves ("self-concept") in light of the leader's influence on their lives. It follows that, if the leader holds out an acceptable vision and the individual chooses to act on the leader's direction toward the ideal, the individual is emotionally engaged in the same goals and is thereby highly motivated to achieve success. In this dynamic, a crisis is not necessary. Success is dependent on the valued traits of the leader and the strength of the relationship between the leader and those around the leader.

The four bulleted characteristics of charismatic leadership likely can trigger the self-concept theory in a clinician–patient relationship with a beneficial outcome. An example is given in Case Study 3.

CASE STUDY 3

Chuck is an NP employed at a satellite clinic in a rural community where he is the sole provider 4 of 5 days each week, with a physician joining him for a half-day in the clinic each week. Chuck is seeing Todd, a generally healthy 40-year-old he has known for years, who is complaining of ankle pain related to an injury that is diagnosed as a sprain. He is providing patient education when Todd interrupts him.

"So, Chuck, I saw you at my friend's father's funeral this week. My friend said you took care of his dad before he died."

Chuck stays to task with his patient education, "Yes, let me finish about you and your ankle. I want you to take it easy with it. . ."

"My friend spoke really highly of you, Chuck. He said you were the best. He said it was because of you that his dad quit smoking."

"Does that make you think about your own smoking habit, Todd?"

"Well, the way my friend put it, you added years to his dad's life when you got him off cigarettes. Sitting at that funeral, it got me thinking. . ."

"That could be a great way to honor your friend's dad, if it brought you to finally letting go of that habit. Do you remember how I told you a while ago about my own journey?"

"How you lost all that weight so that you could climb Pike's Peak?"

"You do remember," Chuck responded. "I did that climb to meet a challenge from my kids."

"And as I remember, you said it was the hardest but best thing you'd ever done."

"Todd, it could be the same for you. I know you can do it. Take the step and quit smoking today. I've got some ideas to help you. Can we talk it over?"

Chuck recognized by his patient's statement about his friend's dad that he was thinking seriously about the dangers of his smoking habit. As he was just at the funeral, Todd was naturally vulnerable in pondering his own immortality. Chuck avoids any scare tactics and responds to Todd's kind flattery by raising the vision of smoking cessation. He then addressed the shared values of his own weight loss with Todd's need to quit smoking. Todd already knew of Chuck's path to reaching his ideal with the unconventional goal of a Pike's Peak climb, and the self-sacrifice required was obvious. Chuck used the opportunity to highlight his own qualities of charismatic leadership to see if Todd would perceive these as shared ideals.

Seeing that Todd was thinking over these values, Chuck reached out to see if they could work together to help Todd reach the goal of smoking cessation. Just as charismatic leaders influence their followers to embrace common values, Chuck was able to help Todd find new meaning to why he should stop smoking. He was able to encourage Todd that, in this moment, he was capable of achieving this goal and that support was available. While this was not a crisis, Todd was especially serious in questioning his smoking habit. These factors all contribute to how charismatic leadership is found to be effective in influencing others to reach a goal.

An interesting factor of influence that can be unpredictable though notable with charismatic leadership is the *emotional contagion*. This social construct refers to how an enthusiastic person can often influence others to be at least more positive if not also to increase their own enthusiasm. In the model of charismatic leadership, the emotional contagion of the leader can be passed to others who find the actions of the leader inspiring. In Case Study 3, it was Chuck's ability to help the friend's father stop smoking that impressed Todd's friend; this was then communicated to Todd, impressing him so much that he voiced it during the office visit.

Dangers of Charismatic Leadership

Lest charismatic leadership be idealized, there are risks to charismatic leadership that deserve clarifying here. These may be particularly dangerous when they occur in patient care. For example, the APP known for her charisma is often optimistic and self-confident, which effectively influences others. However, excessive optimism can obscure the understanding of facts pointing to an undesirable outcome, such as falsely reassuring a patient with terminal cancer that everything is going to be fine. In other charismatic clinicians, the leader may be viewed as never making an error or mistake, so that when by human nature something unfortunate happens, the leader as well as the patient suffer greatly by not meeting the expectations of infallibility. For example, a patient who holds the APP in such elevated esteem but then experiences a failed treatment plan may be highly disappointed, if not resentful. Table 3.3 shows other consequences of charismatic leadership that can lead to poor outcomes if they are not guarded against.

Among these negative consequences, one that has a far-reaching negative impact on both the team and patient outcomes is that *successors fail*. When a leader is identified as charismatic, it is nearly impossible to replace what was considered extraordinary talents of that leader. Some health care teams are

TABLE 3.3 Negative Consequences of Charismatic Leadership

Team members are compromised out of awe

Criticism of team leader is avoided

Team leader is considered "infallible"

Team leader becomes excessively confident

Grandiose expectations are likely to fail

Nontraditional methods may be offensive to some

Successors fail

led by a physician who is famous for a high degree of success in dramatic and specialized care. A team that has success in treating patients for a rare, life-threatening infection, if attributed to the leadership of one doctor, would face extreme disappointment if the doctor departs the team and a patient then fails to recover from this infection. While all should recognize that every infection has different characteristics, the guilt if not blame would be difficult for the remaining health care team if patients who previously overcame the same type of infection had been under the care of the departed charismatic doctor.

For this reason, it is critical that any adulation to an individual APP be quickly passed to the team, which may dilute any sense of individual charisma. If the team holds the vision and values, rather than an individual, then outcomes are not dependent on one person.

TRAITS OF MINDFULNESS

Consider the case studies presented up to this point:

» Susan with the rounding team on rounds (Case Study 1, Chapter 1)

» Pam's emergent referral for John's chest pain (Case Study 1, Chapter 2)

» Mark meeting with Dr. Garza and the orthopedic department director on adding a new surgical device (Case Study 2, Chapter 2)

» Annette and the critical care team evaluating the CABG patient (Case Study 1, Chapter 3)

» Rachel proposing to her superiors a new asthma management strategy (Case Study 2, Chapter 3)

» Todd advising Chuck on smoking cessation (Case Study 3, Chapter 3).

All include an APP who is calm and collected, being astute and shrewd before taking action. Keeping in mind these are fictitious case studies that were created solely for illustrating a feature discussed in the text, each individual seems to possess an almost superhuman ability to interact positively and with a high degree of wisdom.

One may argue that those characters are not dealing with all the issues that the typical APP faces. NPs and PAs are expected to demonstrate mastery over large quantities of ever-changing medical information and associated clinical skills with a full commitment to the pursuit of patient outcomes that rival best practice at national standards. Not unlike many health care professionals, they are asked to sacrifice sleep and give up time with loved ones. In real life, these expectations are typically occurring alongside various stresses, such as financial burdens, poor working relationships, and personal or family health issues. Like many health professionals, they are often facing the profound conflict between healing and human suffering. However, APPs have the added pressure of knowing that every action is up for review and scrutiny to assure that, while they are not physicians, the work completed meets or exceeds the expectations of physician care. One may then conclude that these leadership principles may be unrealistic for many individuals unless they have an otherwise unfettered and perfect life. Only then could a person with an otherwise unencumbered life respond prudently in every single instance when faced with these challenges.

Recognizing that the "perfect life" is not plausible or possible, addressing the potential to develop as a leader over time is the objective. Therefore, for APPs to effectively influence and lead others, they must have an acute awareness of their own environment and an ability to identify appropriate actions, cognizant of potential consequences. This is not a skill that comes naturally.

Life circumstances and time provide the incubator for developing these skills, with the APP mindful of learning from past experience. This learning is more intentional when the APP seeks to practice mindfulness, a learned trait that helps the APP make the adjustments needed to interact wisely with others.

Mindfulness is a collection of mental behaviors and exercises that help a person manage stress and improve personal well-being. Mindfulness begins with an unfiltered awareness of all that is happening in the present moment, such as acknowledging the beep of the ECG monitor, the sensation of one's own breathing, the twitch of the patient's hand, and the glazed stare of the chief resident, all without judgment or reaction. Suspending reaction, if even briefly, helps one uncouple from typical perceptions that the individual holds, often arising from strong beliefs or emotions. Learning to pause, exploring these perceptions, offers clearer discernment. This frames a more compassionate response, staying open to alternative opportunities (Ludwig & Kabat-Zinn, 2008).

Mindfulness doesn't just happen. While identified as a trait of an effective leader, it must be intentionally cultivated. The practice of mindfulness involves mental exercises using self-reflection to help process surrounding stimuli. Engaging mentors or other advisors adds perspective and helps bring order when disorder occurs. Over time, as mindfulness is practiced, it becomes easier to maintain a balanced perspective and avoid overreaction with an improved management of stress.

The opposite of mindfulness are thoughtless reactions that include personal, unrecognized bias. Such unconscious bias is common to all and, until acknowledged, it will influence decisions that more likely favor personal gains or self-centered ideologies.

To explore mindfulness, it is helpful to practice exercises that show the intentional effort required. Here and in later chapters, these ideas and exercises will be shared as examples to be adopted or pursued in the practice of mindfulness.

Improving Patient Outcomes by Mindfulness

Particularly for APP students and professionals, the practice of mindfulness requires one to acknowledge the systematic process of rational thinking common to all health care providers. This cognitive insight functions effectively in making moment-by-moment patient care decisions but may be a barrier to mindfulness, as the focus is on thinking rather than the whole of the human experience. For example, the APP may say, "I'll never get my patient to take this prescription." Perhaps because the patient has refused a prescription in the past, the APP logically assumes the patient will do so again. Such an expressed belief is based on cognitive assumptions from a well-tuned, analytic thought-process common to APPs. Behind this statement may also be feelings and ideologies strongly held by the APP that likely are in conflict with the patient. Perhaps the patient has a long history of non-compliance or even distrust that has previously caused frustrations.

The APP must acknowledge that this belief, albeit logical, becomes an obstacle to the professional relationship with the patient. Gaining a fresh perspective by courage, a positive attitude, and decisiveness, the potential of achieving success with the patient returns. Exercising mindfulness can lead to this renewed perspective.

EXERCISE 3.1 EMBODYING PRESENCE

The University of Massachusetts Medical School offers this exercise as an introduction to the practice of mindfulness.

Perform a brief 2- to 5-minute body scan before getting out of bed in the morning. After the morning alarm sounds, stay for just a short while, creating some space to attend to the body as it wakes up. Starting with the feet, thoughtfully notice all the physical sensations present. Slowly moving upward along the body to the crown of the head, take note of how each part of the body feels, noting any awareness of comfort, stiffness, softness, pressure, discomfort, or other physical sensations.

This exercise helps begin the day with more personal awareness and a clear sense of being present in that moment. The same exercise can be used throughout the day to anchor the current moment in mind. Taking time to notice the body as it responds to life can be processed without judgment. The space created is intended to bring a sense of compassion and gratitude, leading to less stress.

www.umassmed.edu/dio/blog/blog-posts/2016/05/ week-one-10-min-mindful-exercise2

SUMMARY POINTS

1. A range of personality traits have been associated with effective leadership, suggesting there is no one-size-fits-all. In the business/ management world, studies have suggested that of the Big Five Personality Types, extraversion is commonly found in effective leaders. However, selecting a specific personality trait consistently for APPs in health care delivery is less important than the APP recognizing the personalities among the team in relationship to her or his own personality. Recognizing how different personalities can impact others then becomes a tool the leader can use to influence (lead) a patient to better health and guide the health care team to achieve its goals.

2. In ever-changing health care environments, identifying the unique traits of the team members that may contribute to or detract from the team's success is necessary. Every patient and every team is different in inherent strengths and weaknesses. The opportunity for the APP to determine what type of balance between directive and supportive traits will effectively influence the team pinpoints which of four styles of leadership may be most useful: directing, coaching, supporting, or delegating. At the same time, recognizing the developmental stage of the patient or team members in the areas of personal competence and commitment will indicate what style of leadership may be most effective. Understanding the traits of the team will help the APP adjust his or her own leadership style to better meet the needs.

3. Popular leaders often show an uncommon charisma. The personality type often associated with this charisma is extraversion. The APP who may not be an extravert or have a high level of charisma may feel inadequate to the responsibilities of leadership. However, leadership theories suggest that the attribute of charisma is often more defined by the people around the leader; it is not so much what the leader does, but how the people around the leader respond to what the leader does. In this way, the APP has less control of a sense of charisma, as it

stems from those around the APP. In health care, this can be not only a help but also a hindrance. When a clinician identifies individuals who have become strongly committed to her or his own vision or values, a thoughtful response with humility will help guide the patient or team toward the desired goals. If such an attribution of charisma by others leads to overconfidence or overdependence, it brings unhealthy and unproductive relationships. The APP who understands the intrinsic power of charisma may then apply it appropriately, but it need not be a requirement of all leaders.

4. When faced with the challenges of health care delivery, including the wide variety of personalities and talents on various health care teams, the APP finds it daunting at times to maintain a positive and productive attitude. As well, the clinician is human, dealing with personal trials and difficulties common to all. Recognizing the inherent need to manage stress well, the APP leader should be self-aware of effective techniques to personally maintain a balanced perspective to consider alternative pathways when needed to bring success. With this, the APP will more likely hold a positive and productive attitude that presages effective leadership.

REFERENCES

Blanchard, K., Zigarmi, P., & Zigarmi, D. (2013). *Leadership and the one minute manager: Increasing effectiveness through Situational Leadership® II.* New York, NY: William Morrow.

Conger, J. A., & Kanungo, R. (1998). *Charismatic leadership in organizations.* Thousand Oaks, CA: Sage.

Goldberg, L. R. (1990). An alternative "description of personality": The big-five factor structure. *Journal of Personality and Social Psychology, 59*(6), 1216–1229.

Hersey, P., Blanchard, K. H., & Johnson, D. E. (2012). *Management of organizational behavior: Leading human resources* (10th ed.). Upper Saddle River, NJ: Pearson.

House, R. J. (1977). A 1976 theory of charismatic leadership. In J. G. Hunt & L. L. Larson (Eds.), *Leadership: The cutting edge* (pp. 189–207). Carbondale: Southern Illinois University Press.

Judge, T. A., & Bono, J. E. (2000). Five-factor model of personality and transformational leadership. *Journal of Applied Psychology, 85*(5), 751–765.

Judge, T. A., Bono, J. E., Ilies, R., & Gerhardt, M. W. (2002). Personality and leadership: A qualitative and quantitative review. *Journal of Applied Psychology, 87*(4), 765–780.

Ludwig, D. S., & Kabat-Zinn, J. (2008). Mindfulness in medicine. *Journal of the American Medical Association, 300*(11), 1350–1352.

Northouse, P. G. (2016). *Leadership* (7th ed.). Thousand Oaks, CA: Sage.

Shamir, B., House, R. J., & Arthur, M. B. (1993). The motivational effects of charismatic leadership: A self-concept based theory. *Organizational Science, 4*, 577–594.

van der Wal, M., Scheele, F., Schönrock-Adema, J., Jaarsma, A. D. C., & Cohen-Schotanus, J. (2015). Leadership in the clinical workplace: What residents report to observe and supervisors report to display: An exploratory questionnaire study. *BMC Medical Education, 15*, 195. doi:10.1186/s12909-015-0480-5

Weber, M. (1947). *Max Weber: The theory of social and economic organization.* New York, NY: Free Press.

4

CLINICAL LEADERSHIP BEHAVIORS

CRITICAL THINKING QUESTIONS

» **Are there leadership behaviors that facilitate improved patient outcomes?**

» **Do the professional competencies of physician assistants (PAs) and nurse practitioners (NPs) include leadership expectations?**

» **What factors in the health care environment help determine the most effective leadership strategies by advanced practice providers (APPs)?**

» **Does the model of servant leadership fit the APP professions?**

» **What distinctions between transactional leadership and transformational leadership best apply to APPs in guiding health care delivery?**

» **Of the four behaviors associated with transformational leadership, which one works best in the health care environment?**

The appeal of leadership for APPs is the opportunity to create an even more significant impact in the professional role. While seeing patients enjoy better health is gratifying, the reward is greater when the role of the APP is maximized in achieving these goals. Case Study 1 is based on a real-life experience as an example of how utilizing leadership behaviors can powerfully impact others.

CASE STUDY 1

Dylan is an NP working in a rural community in family medicine. He's about to knock on the next patient room door and go in when his nurse, Marcia, stops him.

"You know who you're about to see, right?" she asks.

"It's says on my screen that Marvin is next."

"I know, but do you know who this is?"

Dylan shakes his head and Marcia continues. "This is the guy who lives across the street; the one who drives along Main Street with a pile of middle school boys in the back of his beat-up convertible most evenings. They say he's been in the state pen and likely is just on borrowed time before he returns. That's Marvin."

"I'll be careful," Dylan responds, and Marcia adds more.

"He's also the one who sits on his porch across the street each morning and night, shouting cat calls to the nurses as we walk to our cars from the clinic. He's so rude. I just shudder knowing he's here."

Dylan doesn't miss the genuine resentment expressed.

"Maybe get him out of here. We aren't crazy about him being in the building right now," Marcia concludes and walks away to her next patient.

Dylan enters to meet Marvin. His record shows his age as 52 but he looks over 70 with gray, stringy hair touching his shoulders and framing a haggard, lined face. He's wearing a thin t-shirt wrapped too tight around an obese, heaving chest, panting hard as if he has just sprinted a mile.

With a quick introduction, Dylan obtains the history of a man who has had respiratory exacerbations like this on many occasions over his life. He usually waits them out because he can't afford to be seen, but this time was worse. Dylan's brief examination revealed bilateral wheezing consistent with an asthma flare-up. "Hold on, Marvin; I'll be right back with something."

Dylan went down the hall to the medical samples closet to obtain a bronchodilator inhaler and was returning to Marvin's room when he saw Marcia again.

"You're not giving Marvin a free sample, are you? You give him that and someone else more deserving won't be able to have it," she barked.

THE APP'S ROLE TO TRANSFORM

Case Study 1 is a disease presentation that can be quickly managed by the NP in this acute phase to reach improved health. Dosing the inhaled bronchodilator will bring Marvin quick symptomatic relief. However, this Case Study brings many more significant forces at work between Dylan,

Marvin, and Marcia that hold challenges in effectively managing a mix of chronic disease issues, social implications, and economic burdens. This is where maximizing the APP's role may reach more substantive and positive outcomes, such as curbing Marcia's negative attitude toward lower socioeconomic patients, reaching a more comprehensive management of Marvin's asthma and related morbidities, helping Marvin become more productive in his livelihood, improving the professional relationships Marvin holds with the nursing staff, and guiding the influence Marvin has on the youth in the community in a more positive direction.

Dylan's next actions will affect these desired outcomes. Effective leadership principles as an APP offer Dylan direction toward both effective acute care management and the potential achievement of far-reaching and meaningful health and societal goals. In this way, Dylan's behavior is critical to what will happen next.

CASE STUDY 1 (CONTINUED)

"He needs the inhaler," Dylan tells Marcia, "but I'm going to try something that might help all of us." Marcia rolled her eyes and went on with her work.

Returning to Marvin, Dylan gave him a couple puffs of the bronchodilator and talked with him a bit more, getting more of his history. Seeing that Marvin was beginning to breathe easier, Dylan finished his examination to confirm his initial diagnosis. Marvin was now clearly more relaxed and conversing easily.

"The inhaler is going to help you, and here's the sample and your dosing instructions." Dylan sat down and went over the inhaler use and schedule. "We're going to have to keep an eye on this, Marvin. There's likely more going on that will need some attention. Can you come back in a couple weeks?"

"I appreciate what you did to help me, but I can't afford to come right back."

"I understand, but if we're going to keep you breathing better, it's going to take a little more work. Your next visit will be a courtesy call while we figure out your insurance. It's important that we see you again."

"If you can work that out, sure, I can come back."

"And get back sooner if your breathing gets difficult again."

"I understand. You know, no one has given me this kind of help before. Thanks."

"That's what we're here for, Marvin." They both stood to leave. "But one more thing," Dylan added just before opening the door. "I heard from a nurse here that sometimes you're out there when she's walking to her car from the clinic, and you shout out to her."

"Yeah, I like to joke with the ladies," Marvin chuckled.

"It sounds like, though, that you might push them a little too much." Dylan was firm but stayed friendly. *"They feel like you're teasing them and don't like it. Could you work on that? It would help both you and me around here."*

"I know what you're asking, Dylan. I'll work on it. Thanks again for the inhaler."

Dylan used leadership behaviors in communicating with Marvin, particularly at the end of the visit, which will hopefully bring success. The strategies he engaged include a spectrum of transactional and transformational leadership behaviors.

TRANSACTIONAL LEADER BEHAVIORS

Transactional leadership was explained by James McGregor Burns (1978) as a set of leadership behaviors dependent on an exchange between the leader and follower. Promises by politicians, such as lowering taxes or funding special projects, are classic examples of transactional behavior by a leader. If the followers will cast their votes for the leader, the leader will fulfill the promises. In health care, clinicians routinely use transactional techniques to motivate patients to maintain healthy behaviors, such as issuing a 10-day prescription with instructions to return when it is done to receive additional medicine, or maintaining a diet regime with the intent that it may reduce or discontinue some of the drugs being taken if dietary goals are reached. In these clinical relationships, the clinician will perform an action in exchange for the patient doing what is asked.

There are two categories of transactional leader behaviors (Table 4.1): *contingent reward* and *management by exception* (the latter including passive and active forms). Contingent reward refers to granting a reward based on achieving certain established expectations and is common to health care. Management by exception occurs when the leader waits to only point out performance problems after the fact (passive) or establish rules to prevent possible mistakes (active).

A health care executive who is critical of the team's activities only after monthly patient volume outcomes are not met is managing by exception-passive. After the fact, the executive takes corrective action, perhaps penalizing the team for what has already occurred. If, instead, the executive predicts the end-of-month volume is not going to be met and preemptively rearranges work schedules that make the health care providers see more patients, management by exception-active is in force. Corrective measures are actively taken prior to discovering problems at the end of the month. The contingent reward model would be in effect if the team

TABLE 4.1 Transactional and Transformational Leader Behaviors

Behavior	Description
Transactional Leader Behaviors	
Contingent reward	Granting reward for achievements
Management by exception – passive	Routinely pointing out past mistakes
Management by exception – active	Making rules to prevent possible mistakes
Transformational Leader Behaviors	
Individualized consideration	Personal support and coaching
Inspirational motivation	Casting an appealing vision
Intellectual stimulation	Reasoned, creative thinking
Idealized influence	Exemplifying courage and self-sacrifice

understands that they will receive an award from the executive when the monthly outcomes are met.

In Case Study 1, Dylan used the transactional leader behavior of contingent reward to negotiate with Marvin to return for a follow-up visit by offering it as a courtesy (no-charge) visit. He added a subtle transaction by suggesting that, in view of the kindnesses Marvin was receiving, he stop hassling the nurses. Dylan has little to risk and much to gain by trying this with Marvin.

CASE STUDY 1 (CONTINUED)

The day after Marvin's office visit, Marcia, the nurse, pulled Dylan aside. "What did you say to Marvin?" she asked.

"Why? Did something happen?"

"This morning on my walk from the car, Marvin shouted to me, but what he said was, 'Hope you have a great day. Tell Dylan thanks for all the help.' He waved and that was it.

"What did you do?" Dylan asked.

"I waved back and told him I would tell you. It made my day! After I passed by, I heard him greet two more nurses behind me, wishing them a good day. How did you get him to change?"

As noted in Chapter 3, not always do things go the way a leader plans. However, this true story illustrates how the APP has the opportunity, typically with little notice, to make a positive impact that influences much more than just a person's illness or disease.

There are always potential barriers in the health care environment that are influencing the outcomes, such as the social and economic dynamics shown in Case Study 1. Before further exploring leadership behaviors, these environmental factors are given attention in view of leadership.

SCANNING THE HEALTH CARE ENVIRONMENT

Now more than ever, health care systems must adapt to relatively rapid changes in the external environment. While senior leaders in health care administration across the country are dealing with these issues on a daily basis, the APP must also be alert to the local environment that impacts each individual patient and shapes the direction of all health care teams.

The broad range of external factors includes societal influences, technological advancements, economic challenges, and political variables. On a local scale, examples of these factors may include the opportunities for a community to provide a haven to families from a different culture (social), the expanding services of electronic medical records (technology), the local impact of a recession (economic), and the sway of governmental leaders in funding local health care delivery (political). APPs must stay attuned to these matters if they choose to be leaders in health care. This requires a method to understand the interconnections of various external effects to be able to act on decision making and further planning in light of these influences.

In the business/management sector, the "environmental scan" refers to a formal method of analyzing the external national or global environment, often for the purpose of strategic planning. For the APP, the environmental scan serves as a framework for conceptualizing the impact of external factors that will contribute useful information to decision makers.

STEP/SOS Environmental Scan

Behaviors needed by the APP for a useful environmental scan include routine reading of journals and newspapers, including local and regional news as well as national and international sources. While a more organized scanning process may be employed, the casual, regular review that includes a cross section of resources related to the APP's practice setting and community is often sufficient. For example, the *New England Journal of Medicine*, the *Wall Street Journal*, a specialty medical journal, a professional APP magazine, and a credible local news source may together provide the content needed to alert the APP to significant external changes that might require a response in local health care.

The resources are reviewed to determine signs of change, breaking such cues into four categories:

» Sociodemographic changes (S)

» Technological changes (T)

» Economic changes (E)

» Political changes (P).

These categories of change create a framework of the STEP acronym (Morrison, 1992).

The cues placed in the STEP categories are then scored based on their potential impact using a scale first developed by a 16th-century European historian, Fernand Braudel. Each cue is assigned one of three levels:

» **Superficial or surface occurrences:** such as day-to-day news items (S)

» **Opinions:** representing more deeply held beliefs, values, or attitudes (O)

» **Structural occurrences:** change that is integrated into a formal system (S)

Using the acronym of SOS, these are a cross-cutting measure of the level of impact raised by the change. The STEP/SOS matrix (also referred to as the "Braudel-Wilson system," see Table 4.2) allows the APP to mentally consider a snapshot of external conditions that may impact the health care systems, locally or beyond.

TABLE 4.2 Environmental Scan STEP/SOS Matrix

	Superficial/ Surface	Opinions	Structure
Sociodemographic Changes			
Technological Changes			
Economic Changes			
Political Changes			

The Sociotechnical System

Despite these categorizations, no event or change occurs in a vacuum. Issues placed in the sociodemographic category likely will influence the political landscape, if not the economic landscape. A frequently cited business model pairs the sociodemographic changes with technological changes. The sociotechnical system (STS) is an emphasis found in organizational teams that value the natural human social or relational element in most work environments and the dependence on technology for the tools and techniques to accomplish the work. In this model, an impact on the relational environment can predictably also impact the technology environment, and vice versa (Cummings & Worley, 2015).

The advent of electronic medical records (EMRs) is an example of sociotechnology. The EMR now serves to stand between the clinician and the patient and can either improve the relationship or hinder it. Patients claim that some clinicians are not listening and are more focused on the computer screen. Clinicians may argue that they cannot give the patient the attention deserved because of the details requiring attention in the EMR. Others on both sides would find that the EMR has improved patient documentation and the efficient delivery of health care. No matter the outcome, the technology of the EMR has become an STS, directly impacting the clinician–patient relationship.

CASE STUDY 2

Lauren is the senior PA over nine other APPs at Internal Medicine Specialties, LLC, a multispecialty practice in a suburban area of a large city in the western United States. With five busy clinics throughout the community, the APPs typically staff each clinic for general internal medicine needs. The general internists and some subspecialty internists rotate among the clinics and hospital practice. At the twice/monthly meetings of the APPs, it's become clear that the practice volume is growing, leading to significant stress over work–life balance among the APPs. Despite high satisfaction in their scope of practice and physician support, a couple APPs are considering leaving the practice due to unmanageable patient loads. Lauren and the APP team understand that losing any APPs right now could be extremely difficult from which to recover, and she's decided to bring these concerns to the physician leadership. With the APP team in support, she plans to also present recommendations for what could resolve these concerns.

Lauren's proposal from the APP team includes offering to integrate the APPs into the new telehealth system, combined with hiring a new APP and creating a financial incentive for all APPs based on receipts. In preparing her strategy, she performs an environmental scan using the STEP/SOS matrix. Her findings are shown in Figure 4.1.

		S	O	S
S	Influx of migrant workers locally		Some find seasonal work is trending the same as past years	
T	New telehealth system employed at local hospitals			Greater access to medical consultants if technology functional
E	State unemployment rate rises again	Rise is 0.4%, nominal effect in local community		
P	Governor announces 5% budget cuts to Medicaid			Will bring 5% reduction in planned Medicaid revenue

FIGURE 4.1 Example of STEP/SOS matrix.

She is particularly aware of the governor's recent call for a budget cut in Medicaid reimbursement, which will uniformly impact all clinical services across the state. The current influx of migrant workers across the city is a part of the increased patient volume, and the state's recent unemployment numbers were released showing an upward trend. Lauren has considered the impact of these factors from her environmental scan, as she can expect these will be raised in her discussion with the physician and administrative leadership of the practice.

LEADERSHIP COMPETENCIES FOR APP PROFESSIONALS

The task for Lauren in Case Study 2 can be daunting to any APP. Some might argue that the APP should not have to carry the responsibility of decisions that so largely impact personal employment, the health care delivery system, and the outcomes of patient care. However, it is clear that to be effective in the professional role, the APP must embrace such responsibilities and provide direct leadership to guide these processes. If the professions do not own these roles themselves, these responsibilities will be led by others who are not as familiar with the skills and talents of the APP.

In agreement, chief national organizations representing PAs and NPs call for leadership in the professional competencies associated with each profession. It has become imperative that APPs gain leadership skills in their entry-level training, continuing to develop these skills over their professional careers.

Nurse Practitioner Professional Competencies

The National Organization of Nurse Practitioner Faculties has developed the Nurse Practitioner Core Competencies that include clear support for leadership (NONPF, 2011). The preamble includes a call for increased knowledge, skills, and expertise in "leadership and the business of health care."

Their document identifies nine overarching areas of competency, one of which is titled, "Leadership Competencies." Within this section, there is a list of seven areas of leadership focus, including the following three:

» Assumes complex and advanced leadership roles to initiate and guide change

» Provides leadership to foster collaboration with multiple stakeholders (e.g., patients, community, integrated health care teams, and policy makers) to improve health care

» Demonstrates leadership that uses critical and reflective thinking

Physician Assistant Professional Competencies

The six formal PA competencies developed jointly by the four national PA professional organizations (American Academy of Physician Assistants [AAPA], Physician Assistant Education Association, Accreditation Review Commission on Education for the Physician Assistant, and the National Commission on Certification of the Physician Assistant) emphasize the expectation that the PA possess leadership skills.

One competency of "interpersonal and communication skills" clearly identifies the PA as a possible leader of a health care team or other professional group. Another competency, "professionalism," lists attributes of PA leaders such as a "commitment to excellence" and includes a call to "prioritizing the interests of those being served above one's own." Lastly, the PA competency of "systems-based practice" calls for leadership skills as

PAs "work to improve the larger health care system of which their practices are a part" (AAPA, 2013).

SERVANT LEADERSHIP BEHAVIOR AND APPs

APPs in leadership positions clearly break from the top-down hierarchy of traditional leadership models; this is foundational to servant leadership. The paradoxical title can be misunderstood to suggest that the leader is subservient to others, not unlike how the APP may be mistakenly assigned as subservient in the traditional physician-led order of health care professionals. R. K. Greenleaf developed the original prototype of servant leadership from a fictional character, Leo, in the novel, *Journey to the East* by Herman Hesse (1968). The story tells of a group of voyagers seeking to find their fortune during a magical expedition. Leo is a menial servant who sustains the team on their travels. When Leo disappears later in the story, the group falls into disarray and abandons their journey. The storyteller concludes that although Leo was a servant, he was also the noble, guiding spirit of the group—the leader. This frames the concepts of servant leadership to those who do not dominate or ultimately control others, which readily compares to the role of APPs.

The chief characteristic defining servant leadership is the leader's priority to facilitate the growth and development of the team members above his or her own needs (Greenleaf, 1977). As the team achieves personal goals that better each individual, the collective accomplishments likely have greater success. Servant leadership lacks a definitive construct as there are varying characteristics that have been published to identify behaviors distinctive in this type of leadership (described in Yukl, 2013). The following list of behaviors commonly associated with servant leaders (Barbuto & Wheeler, 2006) includes five factors that also have clear application to APPs:

» **Altruistic calling:** A deep-rooted desire to make a positive difference in others' lives

» **Emotional healing:** A commitment to and skill in fostering spiritual recovery from hardship or trauma

» **Wisdom:** A combination of awareness of surroundings and anticipation of consequences

» **Persuasive mapping:** Influencing others using sound reasoning and mental frameworks to conceptualize greater possibilities

» **Organizational stewardship:** An ethic for taking responsibility for the well-being of the community

Because the health care industry is the largest service provider in the world, it has characteristics inherent to servant leadership (Schwartz & Tumblin, 2002). Chairpersons of departments of medicine in academic health centers are called to adopt a servant leadership model (Feussner, Landefeld, & Weinberger, 2016). The five servant leader factors described here align well for most clinicians as they identify with a calling to medicine, give value to emotional healing, pursue wisdom, practice persuasive mapping in guiding patients to improved health, and actively participate in public health efforts at a community level representing organizational stewardship. In the business model of health care, the qualities of servant leadership are associated with higher patient satisfaction as a key measure of successful outcomes alongside increased provider productivity. Growing provider productivity while respecting the patient's experience of care are best guided by a "put others first" leader model that gives priority to the development of the clinical team members (Trastek, Hamilton, & Niles, 2014).

The PA role shares distinctions with servant leadership (Huckabee & Wheeler, 2008). The five behaviors of servant leadership described here were measured in a population of over 300 PAs (by self-ratings and by ratings from others who observed the PA participants), with each behavior notably higher than as measured in other selected professions (Huckabee & Wheeler, 2011). Appendix 8 includes the Servant Leadership Questionnaire used in leadership studies evaluating health care professionals (Garber, Madigan, Click, & Fitzpatrick, 2009; Huckabee & Wheeler, 2011).

In Case Study 1, servant leadership behaviors were observed in Dylan's actions. Dylan desired to make a positive difference in Marvin's life by both caring for his immediate need and negotiating the return visit (altruistic calling). He sought to help Marcia's personal frustration with Marvin's shouting at the nurses (emotional healing), and anticipated consequences in getting Marvin to stop the catcalls (wisdom). He reasoned with Marvin using a new mental framework for viewing both his asthma condition and his relationship with the nurses (persuasive mapping), and he was resourceful in the distribution of limited medication samples to make a positive impact (organizational stewardship).

TRANSFORMATIONAL LEADERSHIP

Since its introduction in the late 1970s, transformational leadership is one of the more popular styles of leadership across the Western continent. Like servant leadership, it is built on a foundation of values and integrity, seeking to transform people via the pursuit of long-term goals. Different from servant leadership, those being led are asked to transcend their own personal interests for the sake of the organization's goals, and the leader serves as a confident role model to drive these motives. The requirements of the leader have been compared to charismatic leadership with many distinctions in common (Yammarino, 1993). Distinctive to transformational leadership, the leader's priority is helping each member reach his or her full potential (be "transformed") for the benefit of the team.

Four behaviors identified in the transformational leader all begin with the letter "I" (Bass & Avolio, 1990):

» **Individualized consideration:** providing personal support and coaching for the individual to contribute to the goals of the team

» **Inspirational motivation:** casting an appealing vision that resonates with the individuals toward reaching the goals of the team

» **Intellectual stimulation:** reasoning with individuals to think differently and creatively about the best path to the team's goals

» **Idealized influence:** setting an example of courage and self-sacrifice to mobilize individuals to be diligent and dedicated to the team's goals

These four behaviors are in no particular order and may occur individually or may be mixed. The leader is not required to possess all behaviors in the transformational leadership model.

The behavior of idealized influence has received attention as being comparable to charismatic leadership. Similar to the trait of charismatic leadership, idealized influence may be an attribution that members make about the leader or base on the actual behavior of the leader. However, in transformational leadership, idealized influence is purposeful for reaching the goals of the team, distinct from supporting the leader's personal goals or self-esteem.

When compared to transactional leadership, transformational leadership holds outcomes that are beyond expectations. In transactional leadership, outcomes are negotiated with established endpoints. In transformational leadership, the expectation is that the outcomes are exponentially greater than what individual team members could achieve independently. The transformational leader guides the team members so that their combined, maximized efforts reach a greater potential; the outcomes surpass predictions.

Sources of power (see Chapter 2) are ascribed to transformational leadership. Communicating clearly from the position of expert or information power is highly influential in individualized consideration and intellectual stimulation. Avoiding the overuse or abuse of reward and coercive power likely supports inspirational motivation and idealized influence. Referent power, identified when others find the leader is authentic in upholding shared virtues, holds the greatest application to transformational leadership in clinicians (Gabel, 2012).

Transformational leadership has an intuitive appeal by its uplifting and positive attitude toward leadership while remaining attentive to the

TABLE 4.3 Examples of Transformational Leader Behaviors by APPs in Health Care

Leader Behavior	Example
Individualized consideration	• Helping a team member deal with a personal issue that is interfering with work • Spending extra time to teach a team member a procedure • Meeting personally with a supervisor to explore what obstacles may benefit from the APP's personal attention
Inspirational motivation	• Staying positive when the team faces discouragement • Giving a sincere pep talk to team members that encourages them to persist • Taking the opportunity to challenge the leadership to enhance or expand health care delivery
Intellectual stimulation	• Suggesting new ways to improve on policies or procedures • Finding solutions to nagging obstacles • Bringing credible research to the leadership in support of new avenues of health care services
Idealized influence	• Assuming extra workloads to help the team reach goals • Coming alongside a struggling partner to model how to achieve greater success • Offering to be the first to try something new or take a risk with an unclear outcome

APPs, advanced practice providers.

values of the team (Northouse, 2016). These attributes are consistent with what health care teams are seeking, so that the APP who explores these leadership behaviors may find a good fit. Examples of each behavior consistent with the health care environment of APPs are found in Table 4.3.

CASE STUDY 2 (CONTINUED)

As Lauren prepares her proposal for the internal medicine practice physician leadership, she considers the transformational leadership behaviors that may contribute to her success. It is her hope that that she can bring the practice leadership to retain her PA team, add another APP position, and establish an incentive payment structure for the APPs, despite the challenges she found in the STEP/SOS environmental scan (Figure 4.1).

She reasons that in approaching the physician leadership, individualized consideration is likely not necessary. The physicians are not looking for her personal support and that would likely come across as ingratiation.

She believes inspirational motivation is likely necessary as the physicians may be looking at the same information she found on her STEP/SOS scan with concerns. In light of increasing unemployment in the news and the expected 5% reduction in state Medicaid reimbursement, it would not seem the right time to add a new APP position due to what they would perceive as high costs and lower revenue. She needs to realistically show that the local economy is not as affected by the state's unemployment figures, which has been reported by local economists. Her coup de gras is a creative, expanded application of telehealth that could offset the Medicaid cuts. This telehealth offering would be driven primarily by the PAs. Presenting this telehealth strategy with intellectual stimulation to stir the discussion will foster interest and direction. Similarly, she believes she can reason with the physician leadership on the benefits of a modest APP financial incentive package, asking for 30% of revenues that exceed an individually established target for each APP. This package, coming only from net profits, allows each APP to gain a reward, as the physicians also do when required to work harder with documented increased patient volume and revenues.

She plans to recommend herself in leading this new direction in exploring telehealth, particularly with the rising migrant population that most likely has the most to gain from this greater access to health care. Despite the extra effort and time on her part, she is enthused with the possibilities it offers and believes she has the knowledge base to bring success to the telehealth expansion, indicating the behavior of idealized influence.

Her proposal leads to a decision point where she will commit to a 6- to 12-month transition in greater use of telehealth in return for both the added APP position and the financial incentive for performance of APPs.

Lauren's proposal in Case Study 2 is daunting if not overzealous. However, she is setting goals that likely exceed expectations of the team and has identified behaviors on her part that, if she can carry out, will lead to success, as seen in transformational leadership. Lauren would not call herself a charismatic leader, nor is she an eloquent presenter. However, identifying the behaviors of the four Is of transformational leadership has helped her frame her proposal to achieve what she believes is needed to keep her APP team together and advance the goals of the internal medicine practice.

While not every APP is dealing with the challenges Lauren is facing, it is likely that there are unique challenges ahead for each APP in practice. Seizing these opportunities in view of what transformational leadership behaviors offer may bring greater opportunities to advance health care, increase access to care, and achieve patient satisfaction at lower costs. What is required is for APPs to identify these opportunities and bring them to the table.

SUMMARY POINTS

1. In the day-to-day business of patient care, APPs are intuitively using contingent reward transactional leadership behavior to achieve patient adherence. This sets expectations for what is required of the patient to gain better health and gives the APP the opportunity to reward the patient when those gains are reached. The APP can maximize these leadership skills by intentionally motivating patients to reach these goals using leadership behaviors that fit the individual situation.

2. The national professional organizations of both PAs (AAPA, 2013) and NPs (NONPF, 2011) have clearly established leadership behaviors within the competencies for each profession. Both sets of competencies emphasize the importance of leadership in carrying out high-quality patient care, working in integrated health care teams, and functioning within systems-based practice. This clarifies that as APPs, the leadership behavior is not a preference or an option, but by each profession's own competencies it is a required expectation.

3. With the abundance of external factors influencing the health care arena, the APP must be keenly aware of the impact of societal influences (S), technological advancements (T), economic challenges (E), and political variables (P) on the local, regional, and national practice settings. The process of STEP environmental scanning is one example that can keep the APP knowledgeable about these four major, constantly shifting influences on patient care. Considering these factors in light of their potential, impact may be evaluated by SOS as identifying the impact as superficial (a news item), opinion (effecting beliefs), or structural (bringing institutional change). The APP who maintains such an environmental scan is then able to consider what strategies are necessary to maintain or improve the quality of patient care delivery.

4. Servant leadership holds to several behaviors that align with the APP role. As APPs typically function with a high level of authority in the middle of some type of organizational hierarchy (no matter how loosely defined), this role positions them to help the surrounding team members grow and develop, whether they be the physicians, allied health team members, nurses, patients, or other health care professionals. The five leader behaviors consistent with servant leadership (altruistic calling,

emotional healing, wisdom, persuasive mapping, and organizational stewardship) coincide with the daily responsibilities of the APP.

5. Transactional leadership is commonly practiced in health care settings and can be expected to bring positive outcomes for patient care. Transformational leadership also resonates with many health care professionals by the four leadership behaviors that define it: individualized consideration, inspirational motivation, intellectual stimulation, and idealized influence. Effective transformational leadership reaches beyond transactional leadership in challenging others to maximize their abilities to not just meet expectations but to exceed these expectations. A team being led by a transformational leader then has the potential to make long-lasting and powerful advancements in health care, both for organizations and for patient outcomes.

6. Each of the four transformational leadership behaviors brings unique contributions to the team being led. *Individualized consideration* may be most useful for a team that has members in need of new skills training or individual psychosocial needs. *Inspirational motivation* is called upon when the team is facing difficult challenges or is feeling a loss of morale. *Intellectual stimulation* will encourage a team to look for creative new ways to solve problems or pursue new enhancements. Lastly, *idealized influence* is indicated when the team needs an exemplary role model to bring greater focus and dedication to the achievement of its goals.

REFERENCES

American Academy of Physician Assistants. (2013). *Competencies for the physician assistant profession.* Retrieved from https://www.aapa.org/career-central/employer-tools/employing-a-pa/competencies-physician-assistant-profession/

Barbuto, J. E., & Wheeler, D. W. (2006). Scale development and construct clarification of servant leadership. *Group & Organization Management, 31*(3), 300–326. doi:10.1177/1059601106287091

Bass, B. M., & Avolio, B. J. (1990). The implications of transactional and transformational leadership for individual, team, and organizational development. *Research in Organizational Change and Development, 4,* 231–272.

Burns, J. M. (1978). *Leadership.* New York, NY: Harper & Row.

Cummings, T. G., & Worley, C. G. (2015) *Organization development and change* (10th ed., pp. 414–415). Stamford, CT: Cengage.

Feussner, J. R., Landefeld, C. S., & Weinberger, S. E. (2016). Change, challenge and opportunity: Departments of medicine and their leaders. *The American Journal of the Medical Sciences, 351*(1), 3–10.

Gabel, S. (2012). Power, leadership and transformation: The doctor's potential for influence. *Medical Education, 46*, 1152–1160.

Garber, J. S., Madigan, E. A., Click, E. R., & Fitzpatrick, J. J. (2009). Attitudes towards collaboration and servant leadership among nurses, physicians and residents. *Journal of Interprofessional Care, 23*(4), 331–340.

Greenleaf, R. K. (1977). *A journey into the nature of legitimate power and greatness*. Mahwah, NJ: Paulist Press.

Hesse, H. (1968). *Journey to the east* (H. Rosner, Trans.). New York, NY: Farrar, Straus and Giroux (original work published 1956).

Huckabee, M. J., & Wheeler, D. L. (2008). Defining leadership training for physician assistant education. *Journal of Physician Assistant Education, 19*(1), 26–31.

Huckabee, M. J., & Wheeler, D. L. (2011). Physician assistants as servant leaders: Meeting the needs of the underserved. *Journal of Physician Assistant Education, 22*(4), 6–14.

Morrison, J. L. (1992). Environmental scanning. In M. A. Whitely, J. D. Porter, & R. H. Fenske (Eds.), *A primer for new institutional researchers* (pp. 86–99). Tallahassee, FL: The Association for Institutional Research.

National Organization of Nurse Practitioner Faculties (2011). *Nurse practitioner core competencies*. Retrieved from http://www.nonpf.org/associations/10789/files/IntegratedNPCoreCompsFINALApril2011.pdf

Northouse, P. G. (2016). *Leadership* (7th ed., p. 176). Thousand Oaks, CA: Sage.

Schwartz, R. W., & Tumblin, T. F. (2002). The power of servant leadership to transform health care organizations for the 21st-century economy. *Archives of Surgery, 137*, 1419–1427.

Trastek, V. F., Hamilton, N. W., & Niles, E. E. (2014). Leadership models in health care: A case for servant leadership. *Mayo Clinic Proceedings, 89*(3), 374–381.

Yammarino, F. J. (1993). Transforming leadership studies: Bernard Bass' leadership and performance beyond expectations. *Leadership Quarterly, 4*(3), 379–382.

Yukl, G. (2013). *Leadership in organizations* (8th ed., p. 349). Upper Saddle River, NJ: Pearson.

5
FOLLOWERSHIP

CRITICAL THINKING QUESTIONS

» What can be learned from a patient to help determine the advanced practice provider's (APP's) most effective leadership approach?

» In health care teams, what strategies help APPs balance their role as it fluctuates between being a leader and a follower?

» What can the APP do to help the team be effective in following its leader?

THE PATIENT AND LEADERSHIP SUCCESS

It is clear that in the dyadic relationship between the APP and the patient, the patient's commitment to follow the direction of the APP is critical for the best health outcomes. The entire relationship is built on the patient being willing to receive the advice and be guided by the APP. If a patient is unwilling to follow the advice of the APP, it is typically time for the patient to find a different health care provider. It is an unhealthy relationship, at risk of future liability.

This demonstrates the important role the patient holds in the relationship. In similar ways, any person at the receiving end of leadership has a vital stake in defining the effective leader. If the follower (here, the patient) does not seek to follow the leader (the APP), the leader will not be successful. One may argue then that the entire success of a leader hinges on the response of the follower. Therefore, the study of followership is critical to understanding leadership.

PATH–GOAL LEADERSHIP

The path–goal leadership model was among the first to give specific attention to followers. Its foundation is determining what best motivates followers (House, 1971), and this principle applies to APPs seeking to motivate patients toward healthy behaviors. While no patient would desire to be called a "follower," the path–goal leadership model is best explained using these terms of "follower" and "leader," the latter referring to the APP's role.

Using four distinct leadership styles designed to best motivate certain types of followers, the path–goal model appears similar to the situational approach to leadership presented in Chapter 3. The distinction is that the situational model of leadership uses the follower factors of commitment level and competence level to determine effective leadership strategies. In path–goal leadership, the characteristics of followers are not as limited and reflect a more holistic view of each follower, which is then related to the leadership styles that best serve to motivate followers. The four path–goal leadership styles (House & Mitchell, 1974) are described with further details presenting follower types in Table 5.1:

» **Directive leadership:** The leader gives clear instructions to the follower, with details on expectations and timelines with clear rules. The APP using directive leadership would address a single course of action for treatment or behavioral change for a patient, giving explicit directions and expect close follow-up to be sure that goals are reached.

» **Supportive leadership:** The leader focuses on creating a friendly relationship with the follower, attentive to individual circumstances and follower well-being with a goal of a satisfying work environment. The APP using supportive leadership would build patient rapport, be approachable, listen well, and give attention to the psychosocial needs of the patient in pursuing improved health outcomes.

» **Participative leadership:** The leader seeks the follower's opinion and input, being sure to arrive at decisions together. The APP using participative leadership would offer options to the patient and obtain the patient's suggestions and ideas in determining next steps toward health goals.

» **Achievement-oriented leadership:** The leader seeks a high standard of excellence, challenging the follower to consistently improve performance, confident in reaching the highest levels. The APP using achievement-oriented leadership would set a high bar for the patient to practice healthy behaviors, expecting that the patient is fully capable of doing so.

Determining the appropriate leadership style is based on characteristics of the followers. Path–goal leadership recommends that the leader

TABLE 5.1 Path–Goal Leadership Styles With Follower & Patient Characteristics

Path–Goal Leadership Style	Follower Characteristics	Patient Characteristics
Directive leadership	Needs structure, adherent to directions	Respects clinical authority, desires clear treatment orders
Supportive leadership	Desires being nurtured, seeks relational moments when tasks are mundane	Needs to be heard and understood, likely talkative
Participative leadership	Independent, tolerates ambiguity, desires control	Desires sound advice with negotiation in treatment options
Achievement-oriented leadership	Welcomes challenges, desires to excel	Can-do attitude, rises above defined obstacles

understand what best motivates the followers, offering potential characteristics that may shape their individual motivational influences. These include the follower's *preference for structure* (providing certainty, avoiding ambiguity), *need for affiliation* (requiring a friendly, supportive environment), *desire for control* (being in charge or tolerating risks that include luck or chance), and *self-perceived skills* (level of self-confidence), among others.

This model becomes somewhat complex in determining these qualities in the followers related to the tasks before them. It requires identifying and removing barriers to the follower's success. The intricacies of motivation that followers experience when being led extend across a continuum from purely altruistic, internal factors to the opposite extreme of completely extrinsic, reward-type factors. The model has grown to include additional leadership styles that apply to working with groups, networking with others, and values-based leadership (House, 1996), all of which readily apply to the organization and team but has less direct application to direct patient care.

In the following Case Study, an APP has the morning schedule of established patients whom she knows well. She tailors her approach to each patient based on these four path–goal leadership styles.

CASE STUDY 1

Brittany is an family nurse practitioner, working in a rural family medicine clinic and begins her day seeing Mr. and Mrs. Plimpton, an elderly couple routinely scheduled for monthly blood pressure checks as his can be labile. Married over 50 years, they make a habit of always coming to the clinic together, even if only one of them has an appointment. A doctor who recently retired saw them for years. Brittany has assumed their care and been accepted warmly.

Brittany hears about the Plimptons' grandchildren's enjoyable recent visit while finding that Mr. Plimpton's blood pressure is elevated again. This is not surprising, and he is expected to respond well to adjustments in the dosing of his three prescribed antihypertensives. After the evaluation, Brittany writes out the new dosing adjustments, knowing that Mrs. Plimpton will see that her husband follows her directions to the letter. They mention that they will be back for a recheck in 2 weeks before Brittany can suggest it. There's never a question from the Plimptons; their compliance is refreshingly consistent.

Next, Brittany sees Freda for her routine follow-up of diabetes and obesity. Freda is in her 50s, happy-go-lucky and a bit forgetful. Today her HgbA1c is acceptable at a high normal, but her weight has gone up 4 pounds since her last visit. Brittany visits about Freda's diet and exercise regimes and hears of no challenges accounting for today's weight gain. Brittany speaks firmly with Freda, reinforcing her previous success in weight loss on the prescribed diet and setting a 4-pound goal (challenging but realistic) for next month's visit. Freda first exclaims that it will be too hard, but by the end of the visit, Brittany has her talking with new resolve that she can and must reach this weight loss goal to gain control of her diabetes and overall health.

After Freda comes Jorge complaining of hip pain, likely a flare of his arthritis. Jorge is elderly but independent, never married ("no woman can stand to live with me") and stays active for his age. After her examination confirms the acute symptoms from his chronic disease, she offers him the options of a steroid joint injection, a change in his oral NSAID, or a referral to an orthopedist for possible joint replacement. Jorge tells of how he has already thought through the same options himself. He's wondering if it's time to see the surgeon. Brittany sets him up with a referral. Jorge says he'll tolerate the pain for now, and he'll be back to talk over with Brittany what the surgeon recommends.

Alfred is next with an exacerbation of his chronic bronchitis. She asks if he took all of the antibiotics given last month for the same symptoms. He sheepishly smiles, saying that he felt better after a couple days so stopped it to save the rest for later. He's been taking it now the last couple days and it's not helping. Brittany knows Alfred is a lonely man and always seems to perk up after he comes for a visit. After examining him, she diagnoses a secondary infection worsening his chronic bronchitis. She talks to him about antibiotic resistance and the importance of taking his medicines as prescribed. Adjusting his COPD medications, she begins a new antibiotic. She talks a bit more with Alfred, finding out about an upcoming trip to visit his son, and she uses that to encourage him to do all he can to get well.

She hears about plans to visit a zoo as part of the trip. She makes it clear that she wants to hear all about it when he comes back. Alfred leaves after expressing to Brittany how much he appreciates her taking time to listen to his stories about his family.

In Case Study 1, Brittany has sized up the patients she knows and has used different leadership styles based on each of their motivational needs. With the Plimptons, she uses directive leadership to be prescriptive, expecting that with clear directions they will be diligent to carry out her adjusted medicine dosages. She finds Freda lacking motivation as she slips in her weight goals. Brittany reestablishes the targets, pushing Freda to return to her former drive to adhere to her diet and continue to lose weight, expecting a 4-pound loss in the next month. This would represent achievement-oriented leadership. With Jorge, she uses participative leadership, knowing that Jorge's independent nature works best when he can choose from options. And with Alfred, she works at supportive leadership, using a friendly and communicative approach to motivate him to be more compliant in completing his antibiotic therapy.

Path–goal leadership offers APPs leadership skills to help patients stay motivated toward healthy behaviors. In every patient encounter, effective leadership skills guide the patient toward the best health outcomes.

APPs LEADING TEAMS

The challenge can be greater when this leader–follower relationship is taken beyond the clinician–patient environment. In the older, traditional medical team hierarchy, nursing and allied health members understood themselves as followers and physicians as leaders. In today's integrated health care teams, these roles are often more blurred. Nursing and allied health members do not and should not perceive themselves as followers. Nor do physicians perceive APPs as followers. The physician may be absent, so the role of leader is not consistently clear or may be shared. Relationships in the team do not necessarily represent the hierarchy of leader–follower. In this current leadership climate, other models of leadership are needed that give clarity to the role of today's team members. The path–goal leadership styles described earlier may not fit as well in these team-based interactions.

Today's APP is often assigned a role as an agent of the physician, so the APP is positioned to lead the health care team. The team members, accustomed to the physician leader, will view this change as significant. Some will welcome it, and some may doubt the ability of the APP to lead. The APP will learn this quickly as the skills and knowledge of the team are invaluable to the team's success. Keeping the team together is the priority.

If the APP assumes a dominant leadership style, it raises the risk that some team members will feel less valued and may cause them to withdraw.

Similarly, in today's progressive health care systems, there is a less-defined hierarchy between physicians and APPs. APPs find that physicians likely respect their knowledge and skills and are comfortable delegating to them traditionally physician-led leadership tasks in health care teams. While the APP still views the physician in a position of authority, the relationship between the APP and the physician is often more collaborative with shared knowledge, shared skills, and shared responsibilities for patient care.

In this chapter, the leadership styles presented thus far are in the context of the clinician–patient relationship. The focus of this chapter will now transition to exploring the role of the APP integrated into the health care team of physicians and other health professionals.

LEADER–MEMBER EXCHANGE THEORY

The basis of the *leader–member exchange* (LMX) *theory* avoids focusing on either the leader or the follower, but explores the interaction *between* the leader and individual members of the team. This is suited well for study in health care teams to help leaders understand distinctions in the individual relationships with each team member.

The original premise of LMX theory suggested that members fall into one of two groups, either in-group or out-group (Dansereau, Graen, & Haga, 1975). In-group members have stronger relationships with the leader, and those members serve in additional capacities and receive more information and feedback from the leader. Tasked with maintaining the status quo, the out-group members are not involved in extra projects nor receive extra attention from the leader. The "out-group" is not meant to be a disparaging term and should not indicate any sense of discrimination; those members are treated fairly and are content to do their jobs without any extra demands. However, the in-group members have advantages such as opportunities to develop in their roles with the leader intentionally investing time and effort into their individual growth. In an industrial assembly line or other factory labor, this distinction between in- and out-groups fits well. However, LMX theory has evolved to emphasize the value of in-group relationships, which better fits today's health care teams.

In the 1990s, LMX measured how in-group members were more productive, had improved job satisfaction, and greater organizational commitment (Gerstner & Day, 1997; Graen & Uhl-Bien, 1995). Not surprisingly, those in the out-group resented in-group members, perceived as "favorites"

(McClane, 1991). This led to a greater focus on developing leader–member relationships that met the high-quality exchange of the in-group.

For APPs leading health care teams, this means they need to be aware of the tendency to, intentionally or subconsciously, categorize team members by in-group or out-group membership. Assumptions that some allied health or nursing members are merely present to do their jobs while other team members are viewed as being more engaged, and therefore placed in a more favored status on the team, could lead to concerns over fair treatment. The lessons from this more recent model of LMX suggest that the leader should seek to view all team members as potential in-group members. In this way, team members are supported to be more productive, more satisfied, and more committed to the institution according to these research outcomes.

In another study of the LMX model, 69 teams created with five to seven members each were explored for what personality factors were perceived by leaders and members (using the Big Five personality types; see Chapter 3). The most common personality factor that leaders sought in members was extraversion—for example, members who were assertive, enthusiastic, and seeking interaction. This was in contrast to what members looked for in leaders, which fit the agreeableness personality type, representing a leader who was cooperative and trustworthy (Nahrgang, Morgeson, & Ilies, 2009). The reverse did not hold; extraversion in leaders did not influence relationship quality for the members, and agreeableness in members did not influence relationship quality for leaders.

These findings may be helpful to APPs leading health care teams, recognizing that while the APP may seek assertive, gregarious members, those characteristics are not necessarily desirable in the leader as viewed by the members. As well, while the leader is not seeking qualities of agreeableness in the team members, they may expect these from the leader.

Giving Corrective Feedback

The LMX theory sheds light on the relationship expectations between the leader and team members, and how the support of effective relational interactions is integral to a successful team. The greatest threat to this relationship is when a team member requires correction for making an error or is otherwise deficient in completing a task. The risk of medical errors in health care environments continues to be too high, now reported as the third leading cause of death in the United States (Makary & Daniel, 2016). While important emphasis is given to developing systems that can protect against errors, there remains the human element of fallibility that inevitably occurs.

CASE STUDY 2

Jamal is the senior member over four other physician assistants (PAs) in an endocrinology clinic. The PAs gather for team meetings once a week at 6:30 a.m., and the clinic begins to see patients at 7:30 a.m. Howard, employed 2 years with the clinic, has always been notoriously late for the weekly meeting with an excuse of how busy things are at home. Jamal is aware that Howard's late arrivals have more recently occurred unpredictably on one or two other days of the week. Then he is late to see his first patient of the day, often by 10 to 15 minutes, which skews the rest of the day's schedule. Jamal's aware of the stress this brings to the nursing and other support staff, creating a risk for error.

Jamal sets a time to meet with Howard tomorrow and prepares his strategy for this conversation.

In the dyadic relationship, it falls upon the team leader to provide corrective feedback and intervene in high-risk situations to prevent errors. While these are difficult conversations, this should be a discussion focused on the problem with supportive feedback that minimizes the chances of the team members becoming overly defensive or angry (see Table 5.2).

TABLE 5.2 Ten Steps of Corrective Feedback for APPs

1. Address the issue with the team member privately and promptly.
2. Objectively define the concern as directly related to the undesired outcome.
3. Be self-aware of unconscious bias.
4. Clearly explain the adverse impact of the team member's actions.
5. Avoid expressions of anger or rejection.
6. Together explore factors contributing to the problem.
7. Ask the team member to suggest corrective measures.
8. Agree together on corrective measures, supporting the team member to reach success.
9. Determine action steps and timeline to reach desired outcome.
10. Recap the discussion and establish a reassessment plan.

APPs, advanced practice providers.

1. **Address the issue with the team member privately and promptly.**

   The inherent difficulties in giving corrective feedback make the leader prone to postpone it. However, in respect to the rest of the team, when a problem occurs, it is best to address it promptly. Waiting often only allows the problem to escalate, raising more emotion on the part of both parties. Priority should be given to meeting with the team member privately, which shows respect for the member and allows the leader to better control the environment and the conversation without interruption.

2. **Objectively define the concern as directly related to the undesired outcome.**

   Particularly if the leader has not observed the behavior in question, it is important to present the information of concern as either a known fact or a perception that the leader has confirmed with a high degree of truth. The leader should be knowledgeable about the timing and frequency, the severity, and the setting around the problem. While it is informative to report the direct source who raised the concern, there are times that confidentiality needs to be maintained.

   In Case Study 2, Jamal establishes a time within 24 hours to meet one on one with Howard. This affords Jamal time to be sure of his information and to define the concern clearly to himself before visiting with Howard, addressing steps 1 and 2.

3. **Be self-aware of unconscious biases.**

   The leader should be self-aware of the tendency to assign blame or make other hasty judgments based on hearsay or unsupported perceptions, collectively known as "unconscious biases". The leader should avoid immediately assuming that a problem is due to insubordination or incompetence.

   Personally, the leader should recognize various forms of unconscious bias, as these present subtly ("unconsciously"). Cognitive bias (thought patterns that affect judgment) and affective bias (feelings that interfere with judgment) are common to the human capacity (Croskerry, Singhal, & Mamede, 2013). Premature judgments rely on unconscious biases, such as when others determine the problem's source, based on previous unpleasant interactions or stereotyping the member. A leader's fatigue or high stress can lead to unfair judgments. The leader is responsible to be personally aware of these biases and approach the discussion independent of their influence.

As Jamal in Case Study 2 considers the information he has received and his own frustrations with Howard's previous tardy appearances at the team meetings, he needs to be determined to hear Howard's response with an open mind when his concerns are raised.

4. **Clearly explain the adverse impact of the team member's actions.**

   Address the specific behavior with accurate examples. Vague criticisms ("You're lazy") or exaggerations ("You're always late") are argumentative and unclear. After briefly explaining perceptions about the behavior, tie the concerns to the real or potential adverse outcomes that hold a deleterious effect.

5. **Avoid expressions of anger or rejection.**

   With an awareness of unconscious biases, the leader can maintain a professional tone. The problem should be addressed calmly, avoiding any overreaction to expressed anger or frustration. Criticizing the person defeats the purpose. Staying above reproach in valuing the member and the leader's desire to find an equitable solution should be preeminent. Reaching this point without controversy, the remaining five steps will likely unfold in the most helpful way.

   Jamal in Case Study 2 was able to report that by records and documented patient feedback, Howard's late morning starts were recurring on specific days, and that Jamal had seen a recurring issue of timeliness at the weekly meetings. While Howard did not speak in defense, Jamal could see that Howard was embarrassed and avoided belaboring the concerns. He said his chief concern was that hurrying to catch up throughout the day put Howard and his staff at risk of a patient error that could have a serious outcome. This was why he wanted to bring it to Howard's attention before it reached that point.

6. **Together explore factors contributing to the problem.**

   Listening to the member's response to the problem is essential to confirm situational factors and avoid incorrect assumptions. Tolerate valid excuses at this point; acceptance of blame is not necessarily the goal, even if it is obvious. The process of self-evaluation by the member may require time beyond this discussion to appreciate the gravity of the situation. Admitting mistakes or carelessness is difficult and best comes from the member after self-reflection if time is not critical. Keep the focus on the specific behavior rather than sweeping statements of failure.

7. **Ask the team member to suggest corrective measures.**

   Having the team member describe corrective actions implies responsibility for correcting the behavior. Before stating the leader's own suggestions (which likely have been thought out), the member should contribute ideas that often are the same or similar to what the leader has already considered.

Jamal asked Howard, "What do you think can be done to avoid this from happening again?"

8. **Agree together on corrective measures, supporting the team member to reach success.**

The leader can endorse the best corrective measures raised, and the member should own the responsibility for correction. Unless there are issues that require the leader to engage the situation, it is best to give the team member charge over the next steps of correction. The leader can use this time to affirm the member, who likely is discouraged and deserves support. Genuinely stating the strengths and better qualities of the member builds confidence that success will be reached.

9. **Determine action steps and a timeline to reach the desired outcome.**

The leader's role is to ensure that corrective actions are taken. To be clear, the leader should restate, if not write down, the action steps required. This should include specific performance expectations. Establish a sufficient length of time for the member to make necessary adjustments or corrections, with an expected follow-up visit. The leader should state that if the undesired behavior persists, further actions would be necessary, though these do not need to be explicit unless this is a repeated issue that requires more serious or formal consequences. Schedule another meeting now to occur at the end of the timeline to visit about progress and determine if other obstacles were uncovered, with the expectation that the member will be affirmed if goals are reached.

10. **Recap the discussion and establish a reassessment plan.**

The meeting should conclude with the leader able to express appreciation for what has hopefully been a frank and honest discussion. If the visit had any trouble spots or unresolved conflicts, the leader should note these and address how to solve them, which may simply require time for emotions to heal. The leader should stay in control of the meeting's conclusion with assurance that the member understands the expectations and the measures used to confirm that the corrective actions are applied. The leader should ask if there is anything else that needs discussion or if the leader can do anything further to support the member. If the member has nothing else to say, the leader may end this meeting, asserting that the next meeting should go better.

In Case Study 2, Howard reported that getting out of the house with the needs of his kids and wife is difficult each morning and placed fault on the home front. However, he reported that he could get up earlier in the morning and try to organize his family to be more responsible with their needs to allow him to leave the house on time. He recognized that the patients and staff were depending on him to be on time and realized the distress caused by his late arrival. Jamal affirmed Howard's suggestion to arise earlier and establish a plan at home to leave on time. He noted that Howard was a good husband and father, and getting up a little earlier would likely help him accomplish much with less stress at home. Howard agreed. Jamal set a meeting to revisit these concerns in 1 week, with an expectation that there would be no further late arrivals after today. Howard said he would do his best. When asked if there was anything else to discuss, Howard said all else was fine. Jamal reminded Howard that he was available to help and they would plan to visit again in 1 week.

These 10 steps offer a strategy to address a specific focus on skills or behaviors that miss the mark. When this corrective feedback does not yield a positive outcome, or when the issues are more serious, such as negative attitudes or more severe lapses in judgment, a more intensive level of correction may be necessary and will be discussed in the next chapter.

ADAPTIVE LEADERSHIP

Adaptive leadership offers a model focused on the work of the members in relation to the activities of the leader. The emphasis is on how to motivate and mobilize the team members, which requires the leader to help the team adapt to varying circumstances to reach their goals (Heifetz, 1994). There are no traits or behaviors specific to adaptive leaders.

Adaptive Leadership and Complexity Leadership Theory

More recently, adaptive leadership has been included as one of three leadership elements in the Complexity Leadership Theory (Uhl-Bien, Marion, & McKelvey, 2007). Today's environment presents turbulent social influences, such as the economy or politics, creating external complexities. As the relational organization of today's teams move away from the hierarchical leadership model, the complexity leadership theory suggests three types of leadership processes (administrative, adaptive, and enabling) that together facilitate progress for an interactive organization in this dynamic environment.

The *administrative leadership* component involves the formal leadership roles. The *adaptive leadership* component addresses the varying levels of team knowledge and influence with fluctuating needs and ideas. *Enabling leadership* guides the process of engaging people in the necessary interactions.

In the mix of challenges in health care delivery, the leadership activities associated with adaptive leadership are useful in addressing multiple facets of an intricate health care system when the issue is complicated. For example, dealing with the multiple challenges a health care team faced when navigating a patient's transition to hospice care represents a place for adaptive leadership. Family dynamics, facility environments, ethical considerations, financial implications, medical treatment decisions, and tailored health professional roles all require attention in moving to the palliative care of hospice, and often the demands occur simultaneously.

Adaptive Leadership Activities

Six leader activities (Heifetz, Grashow, & Linsky, 2009; Heifetz & Laurie, 1997) guide the health care team to surmount challenges and make decisions in facilitating a desired outcome (Table 5.3).

TABLE 5.3 Activities for Leading Health Care Teams in Adaptive Challenges

Leader Activity	Description	Application
Get on the balcony	Step away from the chaos to gain clarity	Avoid reactive decisions; get away from the activity to think through the challenge using scenarios
Identify the adaptive challenge	Challenges that trigger an emotional response likely require attention by the team	Separate issues that can be solved by the leader's decision from those that need to be solved collectively by the team
Regulate distress	• Establish a safe work environment • Manage conflict • Regulate personal distress	• Create a culture of honesty and transparency • Ask, "What would you want to see done to resolve this?" • Practice MBSR

(Continued)

TABLE 5.3 Activities for Leading Health Care Teams in Adaptive Challenges (*Continued*)

Leader Activity	Description	Application
Maintain disciplined attention	Redirect the team when it shifts from needed change	Establish small "wins" to keep team on track
Give the work back to the people	Pull back directive leadership so team makes progress itself	Ask, "As this is the team's work, what do you think we should do?"
Protect leadership voices from below	Respect the value of minority voice criticisms	Find a way for fringe members to engage with the team

MBSR, mindfulness-based stress reduction.
Source: Adapted from Heifetz and Laurie (1997).

1. **Get on the Balcony**

   This metaphor speaks of the need for a leader to step away from the dance floor and stand on the balcony to envision the big picture. The leader finds that being away from the noise and chaos of a situation allows a perspective that brings clarity for what the team needs to be effective in the midst of the challenging environment.

2. **Identify Adaptive Challenges**

   Not all challenges are adaptive. Some are technical, such as schedule designs, use of technology, or simply financial issues solved by an authority role. Adaptive challenges, however, are layered with individual opinions, values, and other sources of conflict. If there is a challenge that triggers any type of emotional response, it is likely an adaptive challenge. Various degrees of coping skills are needed among all the parties involved. The leader should not authoritatively solve the problem; it is best to have solutions come from the individuals affected. The leader identifies the challenges that are adaptive to determine the support needed to mobilize everyone forward (which may be that the leader gets out of the way).

3. **Regulate Distress**

   Because of the inherent uncertainty in change, particularly change that impacts values and beliefs, distress within adaptive challenges is common. The leader needs to control the team's response to the inevitable distress, which can be used productively, helping maintain focus without being overwhelmed. Adaptive leadership offers three areas of focus for the leader: the environment, conflict management, and regulating personal distress.

The environment

The leader is responsible to establish a work environment that supports safely engaging difficult problems. This may include the physical location, communication methods, established procedures and processes, and the relational culture of the team. When the environment is stable and supportive, the team can better attend to specific issues leading to effective decision making.

Conflict management

Note that the term "conflict resolution" is *not* used here. While conflict is inevitable, resolution is not always possible. If adaptive change is to occur, the leader can anticipate conflict and should not ignore it. An early question to pose to those involved in the conflict is, "What would you want to see done to resolve this?" Often, those involved in the conflict need only to be heard and understood, not expecting a "fix." If there is a specific request to take action, that can be considered. However, the answer may be, "I just needed to get that off my chest. We can go back to work now."

Conflict is unpleasant, but not necessarily unhealthy. That members find a safe environment in which to be transparent and speak honestly about doubts or disagreements is often a productive phase that brings growth and refines the team's focus on the goal. The APP should not fear conflict and needs to stay open to facing contrary thinking so that everyone learns from it.

Regulating personal distress

Stress accompanies adaptive change, and the leader will not be immune. There will be those resistant to change (see Chapter 9, Change Strategies in Health Care). The leader will experience tension in making decisions that lead the team forward. This is not abnormal; many leaders enjoy facilitating change, if not thrive on it. However, too much stress can become unproductive and unhealthy. Adaptive leaders must have the emotional capacity to handle conflict and tension. This requires self-confidence and an internal measure of the degree of anxiety experienced in the workplace, personally, and in relationships or family members outside of the workplace. The cumulative impact of stress on multiple fronts often triggers breakdowns or disaster.

Practicing mindfulness (introduced in Chapter 3) can help leaders regulate personal stress. A study of over 300 second-year medical students divided into groups who received training in mindfulness-based stress reduction (MBSR) methods compared to a control group that received training in complementary/alternative medicine without specific training in mind–body techniques (Rosenzweig, Riebel, Greeson, Brainard, & Hojat, 2003). Over a 10-week intervention period, those receiving MBSR training (N=140 students) reported significantly lower scores in tension-anxiety and confusion-bewilderment and significantly increased scores in vigor-activity as compared to the control group. The fatigue-inertia scores were stable in the MBSR group, while the control group measured a significant increase over 10 weeks in comparison. The types of MBSR exercises used in this study are shown in Table 5.4.

Being sure to avoid dependency on drugs or alcohol, the leader is responsible to have a collection of self-selected tools for managing stress and avoiding overload. The use of mindfulness techniques may be among the tools of value.

4. **Maintain Disciplined Attention**

When facing adaptive challenges, the team is tempted to avoid conflict and choose easier routes than the necessary change. Signs that the team is moving away from change are when team members begin to cast blame, speak negatively against the institution, or ignore the problem. The effective leader will be alert to these tendencies to facilitate more focused attention to necessary direction of effort. This may result in targeting short-term goals for accomplishment, using contingent reward strategies, so that the team can experience some small "wins" along the course.

5. **Give the Work Back to the People**

In the midst of the aforementioned four adaptive leader activities, APPs may find themselves stepping in with greater involvement than typically expected on a health care team. When the team challenges are difficult, the strong leader will feel the need to give direction and provide direct oversight to be sure the team stays on track. However, this may also lead the team to become overly dependent on the leader, or the team may just step aside to let the leader take over. The leader needs to recognize opportunities to sit back and have the team members work together to solve a challenge, even if it takes longer or becomes more complicated. The benefit to the team's morale and later effectiveness when facing challenges that are more difficult is worth it.

This is a cornerstone of adaptive leadership: *The work of the team remains the focus*. The adaptive leader monitors when his or her leading is too strong. When asked by the team for a leadership decision, the leader should respond, "As this is the team's work, what do you think we should do?" When the team is empowered to make decisions together, the outcomes are more readily achieved.

6. **Protect Leadership Voices From Below**

   In most teams, there are those who feel marginalized; the team's direction is not necessarily where they wanted to go. These members are likely to be in the out-group under the LMX theory of leadership, as they are doing the tasks as requested but do not feel engaged. These fringe members may also be antagonistic to the team's advancement. Leadership may find it convenient to ignore these members to avoid upsetting the balance of the team's progress. However, these members are not expendable. Though their actions may be disruptive, protecting these voices helps the leader refine the team's goals and direction. The leader should find some degree of value in the opposing opinions. When their interests are recognized, these members will be more likely to engage in the process.

   Appendix 9 includes the Adaptive Leadership Questionnaire to assess these six leadership components in the APP leader.

TABLE 5.4 Mindfulness-Based Stress Reduction Exercises

MBSR Exercise	Description
Body scan	Moving from toe to head, focus on each part of the body to experience feeling (see Exercise 3.1)
Breath awareness	Focus on the flow of air in each breath, noting the rise/fall of the chest and related sensations of breathing
Mindful stretching	Focus on stretching and relaxing muscles across the body, using slow movements with individualized end points
Eating meditation	Think about food about to be eaten; during ingestion note the texture, individual tastes and smells, etc.; analyze the mind's response by the degree of pleasure, satiety, and satisfaction
Walking meditation	Take a slow walk in a peaceful, quiet place, aware of the movement of each foot and arm, sensing aspects of the natural environment, permitting the mind to wander
Mountain/lake meditation	Step away to imagine the majesty of a mountain, loveliness of a lake, etc.; focus on all the elements, large and small, that contribute to the imagery; seek to personalize the most pleasurable elements (peace, clarity, beauty, etc.)

MBSR, mindfulness-based stress reduction.

Adaptive Leadership in Direct Patient Care

Examining adaptive leadership and its focus on what motivates the team to succeed also correlates well with the clinician–patient relationship. This model, applied to direct patient care, presents the patient as a complex adaptive system. While patients' needs may present as technical challenges, they clearly face adaptive challenges that the APP can help them recognize and navigate. Thygeson, Morrissey, and Ulstad (2010) present the clinical example of a patient with low back pain. Treatment will involve pain control, but the long-term solution is stretching and strengthening exercises to restore function and prevent further disability. While the technical challenge of prescribing appropriate pain medications is in order, the adaptive challenge is the patient's therapeutic exercise and conditioning. The clinician is responsible to facilitate the patient's response to both technical and adaptive challenges. Because adaptive leadership focuses less on the leader's actions and more on the member's motivation toward success, the six principles of adaptive leadership give guidance on patient-centered health care delivery.

Eubank, Geffken, Orzano, and Ricci (2012) recommend adaptive leadership as the curricular framework for family medicine residency programs. They teach residents specific adaptive leadership skills (*get on the balcony, identify adaptive challenges,* and *regulate distress*) to maintain patient-centered care and enhance the clinician–patient relationship for better health outcomes.

Adaptive leadership has application for APPs leading health care teams as well as APPs in patient care. The third front is APPs using leadership skills toward those in positions higher than their own, such as physicians. To explore the use of adaptive leadership activities by APPs in working with physicians, Case Study 3 is presented.

CASE STUDY 3

Julia is the sole PA working in dermatology for a pair of plastic surgeons. Their office has a high volume of both aesthetic procedures and reconstructive surgery. Much of her patient volume is through the medical spa office, while the surgeons are involved primarily in the surgical management. She and her good friend, Thomas, have not seen each other for a couple years and are reconnecting over coffee today.

Thomas is a cardiac nurse practitioner who sees patients at the primary clinic and travels 2 days each week to see patients in satellite clinics. His practice consists of patients needing follow-up and management for hypertension, arrhythmias, or valvular disease. Thomas and Julia trade stories on their experiences and ask for advice from each other.

"*I just don't feel like I'm using all my skills,*" *Julia says to Thomas.* "*The patients we see are usually appreciative, but much of what I do is Botox, medical peels and laser hair removal. I'm just the 'technician' to them. I wish the surgeons would want to use me in some of the surgical work-ups. They get a lot of breast reconstruction patients after cancer, and I think I could really help them. I'm jealous of you, Thomas, it sounds like you're given a lot of freedom.*"

"*Don't be so sure,*" *Thomas responds,* "*I don't think you have it so bad. You always have a doctor available to you in a minute's notice. That's my frustration. When I'm out in the satellite clinic, I too often have a patient with a heart rhythm that won't settle down or a sky-high blood pressure. It's up to me to make a med adjustment, but it's tricky. After tracking down one of the doctors on the video line, I'm not always sure they understand what I'm seeing. Sometimes I wish I could have a position like yours, where you have doctors always on site.*"

"*So have you talked with your cardiologists about it?*" *Julia asks.* "*Do they know you're frustrated?*"

"*I don't want to sound like I'm whining,*" *Thomas says.* "*They give me a great deal of responsibility—I like that.*"

"*That doesn't need to change,*" *Julia replies.* "*I wonder if they'd have some suggestions to keep it working, but could find a clearer path of access to them when you have a question. If I were them, I'd want to be sure to hear your questions and make you feel comfortable. You're valuable to them for traveling to the satellite sites. What do you think they could do to help you better?*"

"*It's like you said. If I knew I could call and ask a couple quick questions without waiting 10 minutes on hold, that would really help my day go better.*"

"*Thomas, you're not asking for much. I think you ought to bring it up. It shows your own commitment to the patients you're responsible for and also strengthens the communication you need with those above you. Who's going to argue with that?*"

"*Thanks, Julia.*" *Thomas responds.* "*And I've got an idea for you. Why don't you ask your doctors if you can help with the surgical patients?*"

"*Tried that,*" *Julia retorts.* "*They said it's most cost-effective to keep me with the aesthetics. You know, it's all about the money.*"

"*I'm not so sure. If they knew you wanted to use more of your PA knowledge and skills, I think they would try to work with you. I wonder if they realize you're this frustrated. I bet there's a way for them to give you more responsibilities in the aesthetics office and let you be involved in some types of patient evaluations and work-ups. Shouldn't it be something you can ask your surgeons about?*"

"*You're doing to me what I did to you, Thomas.*"

"*You suggest I talk to my doctors, I suggest you talk to yours. We just need to go to them with a bit more clarity on what we see as the problem,*" *and then offer a couple solutions. Let's both try it and check back with each other in a couple weeks."*

In Case Study 3, Thomas and Julia both use adaptive leadership activities and recommend the strategies to help each other. Taking time to get together and visit represents the *"get on the balcony"* activity. It allowed both of them to think through their challenges and gain some clarity. They then each helped each other *identify the adaptive challenge.* Julia was stuck on the technical challenges in her medical spa, doing procedures to keep up with the patient volume goals. Thomas was similarly held back by looking only at the technical challenges of being sure he was at the satellite clinic to see patients. Once they each saw past that to recognize the adaptive challenges that would require a discussion with the physicians (exploring how to better utilize Julia's PA education and skills and how to help Thomas more quickly consult on patients), it made more sense to look for a solution beyond just the technical issues. They then both encouraged each other to open up honest discussions with their respective doctors, both examples of the adaptive leadership activity, *regulate distress.* By having honest, transparent discussions, they were open to exploring the question, What would you want to see done to resolve this? While they traded answers, using adaptive leadership they should each now raise the discussion of the adaptive challenges and pose that same question to their doctors. Something may come forth that is comparable to their own solutions.

This dialogue with their respective doctors may backfire, but it is more likely that this will open up a conversation that will bring greater awareness and improved patient care delivery. While there is a risk that it will lead to frustration, it is better to have tried to have the conversation than to just bury the concerns, which is another component of *regulating distress* (regulate personal distress).

SUMMARY POINTS

1. When the APP recognizes that the patient is a complex individual distinct from a certain classification of disease, illness, or injury, then the goal of motivating the patient to wellness comes to clearer focus. While the APP has the keys to medications and referrals for care, the APP has the opportunity to facilitate the patient's own pursuit of improved health habits that can have long-lasting benefits. Therefore, the study of what motivates the individual patient has significant value to the APP to achieve these health outcomes. The path–goal leadership model includes four leadership styles tailored to what may be most helpful to the individual patient needs, including directive, supportive, participative, and achievement-oriented

leadership styles. The adaptive leadership model also targets the patient's needs, distinguishing between technical and adaptive challenges. The adaptive challenges are likely more emotional and require more effort on the part of the patient, but yield a more significant health gain, such as recovery from low back pain that is less dependent on medications and more the result of lifestyle modifications (e.g., exercise and weight loss). Knowing the individual patient's motivational needs will guide the APP on how best to lead the patient to better health.

2. Today's complex environment surrounding health care systems requires health care teams to be nimble and wise in responding to challenges and barriers. APPs are integral to health care teams, able to follow the leadership of administrators and physicians as well as be leaders themselves within health care teams that work together to provide sophisticated, multifaceted health care with technology and advancements never before seen. Leader-member exchange (LMX) theory has shown that team members become highly engaged and productive if the leader is able to help each member individually grow and develop. Team members have a tendency to seek leaders who have a personality trait of agreeableness (i.e., leaders who are cooperative and trustworthy). Because of the frequency of medical errors, leaders must be thoughtful to provide corrective feedback with respect, supporting the integrity of the team while preventing future mistakes. Activities of the adaptive leader model—such as getting on the balcony, identifying adaptive challenges, and regulating distress—all guide the team to overcome obstacles to achieve success.

3. The health care team is seeking a leader who listens. The APP can provide bidirectional influence in encouraging team members to communicate their ideas clearly and help the leaders actively listen to the team's suggestions. Helping the team maintain disciplined attention by creating short-term goals to achieve and engaging the team members in the work without overdependence on the leader all help the team feel empowered to pursue the goal together. When possible, coming alongside fringe members who feel marginalized can help give value to their contributions and further unite the work of the team.

REFERENCES

Croskerry, P., Singhal, G., & Mamede, S. (2013). Cognitive debiasing 1: Origins of bias and a theory of debiasing. *BMJ Quality & Safety, 22,* 58–64. doi: 10.1136/bmjqs-2012-001712

Dansereau, F., Graen, G. B., & Haga, W. (1975). A vertical dyad linkage approach to leadership in formal organizations. *Organizational Behavior and Human Performance, 13,* 46–78.

Eubank, D., Geffken, D., Orzano, J., & Ricci, R. (2012). Teaching adaptive leadership to family medicine residents: What? Why? How? *Families, Systems & Health, 30*(3), 241–252.

Gerstner, C. R., & Day, D. V. (1997). Meta-analytic review of leader–member exchange theory: Correlates and construct issues. *Journal of Applied Psychology, 82*, 827–844.

Graen, G. B., & Uhl-Bien, M. (1995). Relationship-based approach to leadership: Development of leader–member exchange (LMX) theory of leadership over 25 years: Applying a multi-level, multi-domain perspective. *Leadership Quarterly, 6*(2), 219–247.

Heifetz, R. A. (1994). *Leadership without easy answers.* Cambridge, MA: Belknap Press.

Heifetz, R. A., Grashow, A., & Linsky, M. (2009). *The practice of adaptive leadership: Task and tactics for changing your organization and the world.* Boston, MA: Harvard Business School Press.

Heifetz, R. A., & Laurie, D. L. (1997). The work of leadership. *Harvard Business Review, 75*(1) 124–134.

House, R. J. (1971). A path–goal theory of leader effectiveness. *Administrative Science Quarterly, 16*, 321–328.

House, R. J. (1996). Path–goal theory of leadership: Lessons, legacy, and a reformulated theory. *Leadership Quarterly, 7*(3), 323–352.

House, R. J., & Mitchell, R. R. (1974). Path–goal theory of leadership. *Journal of Contemporary Business, 3*, 81–97.

Makary, M. A., & Daniel, M. (2016). Medical error—The third leading cause of death in the US. *British Medical Journal, 353*, i2139. doi:10.1136/bmj.i2139

McClane, W. E. (1991). Implications of member role differentiation: Analysis of a key concept in the LMX model of leadership. *Group & Organizational Studies, 16*, 102–113.

Nahrgang, J. D., Morgesen, F. P., & Ilies, P. (2009). The development of leader–member exchanges: Exploring how personality and performance influence leader and member relationships over time. *Organizational Behavior and Human Decision Processes, 108*, 256–266.

Rosenzweig, S., Riebel, D. K., Greeson, J. M., Brainard, G. C., & Hojat, M. (2003). Mindfulness-based stress reduction lowers psychological distress in medical students. *Teaching and Learning in Medicine, 15*, 88–92.

Thygeson, M., Morrissey, L., & Ulstad, V. (2010). Adaptive leadership and the practice of medicine: A complexity-based approach to reframing the doctor–patient relationship. *Journal of Evaluation in Clinical Practice, 16*, 1009–1015.

Uhl-Bien, M., Marion, R., & McKelvey, B. (2007). Complexity leadership theory: Shifting leadership from the industrial age to the knowledge era. *Leadership Quarterly, 18*, 298–318.

6

LESSONS FROM BAD LEADERS AND FOLLOWERS

CRITICAL THINKING QUESTIONS

» **What can be done if the advanced practice provider (APP) is teamed with a bad leader?**

» **When the team has a member in conflict with the leader, what should the APP do?**

» **What best prevents an APP from becoming a bad leader?**

When asked for a list of bad leaders from history, names surface such as Adolph Hitler, Charles Manson, or Jim Jones. There is no argument that the actions of those individuals led to tragic outcomes without comparison in depravity. A study of the leadership styles exercised in those situations remains an active area of exploration to learn both how things could turn out so badly, as well as learn how a person could lead a group down such a destructive path.

There is, therefore, no mistaking the power of leadership. While effective leadership can guide a team to the greatest of accomplishments, bad leadership can bring the most devastating results.

TYPES OF BAD LEADERSHIP

In the context of the health care environment, there are different forms of "bad leadership" (see Table 6.1). It is of paramount importance that the APP be alert to leadership failure, whether among peers, supervisors,

TABLE 6.1 Bad Leadership Types, Qualities, and Progression

Bad Leadership Type	Breached Leadership	Expected Outcome Without Intervention	Path of Resolution if Bad Leadership Uncorrected
Unethical	Ethical standards	Harm to self or others	Formal investigation, potential prosecution, and/or rehabilitation
Incompetent	Competency in leadership	Slowed or halted progress of team	Progression to ineffective or absent leadership
Disruptive	Constructive behaviors	Harm to self or others	Marginalization or removal of leader, may require investigation
Ineffective	Effective in leading	Slowed or halted progress of team	Marginalization or removal of leader
Absent	Attendant to leadership needs	Slowed or halted progress of team	Marginalization or removal of leader

employers, or in oneself. These most likely fall into some form of breach of the following expectations:

» Ethical

» Competent

» Constructive

» Effective

» Attendant

Unethical Leadership

With clearly defined ethical standards of leadership, breaches are easily recognized. Attaining ethical leadership can be challenging (as addressed in Chapter 9); however, distinguishing unethical leadership need not be as difficult. A leader who is committing immoral or illegal behavior, confirmed by clear evidence, needs correction if not discipline. Examples of unethical behavior that may occur in the health care setting include misuse/abuse of alcohol or drugs, physical or sexual abuse, fraud, embezzlement, or other criminal acts. In such situations, the APP needs to be a part of the solution, not the problem.

The APP who is complicit with an unethical leader (e.g., being aware of the immoral behavior), not only shows a lack of leadership skills but also contributes to a potentially harmful outcome. In such situations, the APP is obligated to report the activity to an authoritative office such as a state board, the human resources department, or the agency administrator. When unsure, it is appropriate to contact the authoritative office to share perceptions and explore issues. While it is uncomfortable for the APP, the authorities are likely to bring clarity and may be waiting for better evidence to support appropriate action.

Incompetent Leadership

Concerns over competence in direct patient care are an issue of malpractice that is beyond the scope of this discussion. However, incompetence in leadership, while hopefully not endangering patient care, can lead to many obstacles and challenges. Its origin may seem innocent, such as promoting an individual with a history of exemplary performance to a leadership position without ensuring there is sufficient education or experience to lead.

The novice leader often values assistance with gaining historical knowledge and guidance. The APP, by position in the upper organizational hierarchy, may offer this support to the new leader without political insult. The partnership formed will advance the team goals and bolster the leader to gain the needed competency. If such a relationship is not possible, the leader likely fits into one of the other categories of bad leaders, such as ineffective, disruptive, or absent leadership.

The APP may be the one in over her or his head in leadership challenges. Being self-aware with an attitude of listening well to others will help maintain an objective perspective. The APP should find a potential partner who can respectfully offer guidance and a historical perspective. Seeking formal training and education may be available in the work setting, and requesting such support is no sign of weakness. Seeking opportunities to grow leadership skills is encouraged and likely supported at the administrative level of the organization. However, the immediate needs before the nascent leader may require some immediate friendly advice. When engaging support from a knowledgeable and respected team member, it conveys the APP's desire to keep the team moving forward.

Disruptive Leadership

Disruptive leadership occurs with any type of leader, but in the health care environment, many have experience with a physician who is a disruptive leader. While effective leadership may require change that brings temporary disorder to the team, the leader should avoid being personally disruptive, adding an increased level of frustration and anxiety within the team. Behaviors characteristic of disruptive leadership are notable for intimidation, angry outbursts, coercive and abusive language, sexual harassment, unnecessary sarcasm, lack of respect for others, and threats to harm others.

The health care environment is dependent on clear communication between the team members; these disruptive behaviors prevent effective communication. The example familiar to many APPs is the surgeon who humiliates a member of the surgical team over an error, perhaps throwing instruments and/or cursing in anger. Suddenly the team rises to a heightened attention. The leader perceives by this response that the outburst worked, resulting in improved performance. Rather, while the team's immediate performance may be improved, they are fractured by the mixed emotions of consternation, sympathy for those shamed or offended, and general frustration. The result may lead to errors, cover-ups, and adverse patient outcomes.

A study of 102 hospitals associated with Veterans Health Administration (VHA) West Coast (Rosenstein & O'Daniel, 2008) revealed the magnitude of disruptive behaviors in this sample. A 22-item survey was completed by 4,530 participants; 21% were physicians, 63% were nurses, and 15% did not self-identify. Over half of the physicians and 88% of the nurses reported witnessing disruptive behavior by physicians. Two-thirds of the respondents reported that the disruptive behavior led to adverse events, with 72% of those associating it with patient mortality.

The occurrence of this high rate of physician disruptive behavior caught the attention of The Joint Commission, the accreditation body for most health care organizations and programs in the United States. In 2009, The Joint Commission sought to establish a "culture of safety" at all hospitals by requiring a code of conduct that defined acceptable behavior. Intended to address disruptive behaviors, some physicians objected that their own strong advocacy be misinterpreted as disruptive. The Joint Commission standards (LD.03.01.01) were updated again in 2012 to recommend policies and procedures addressing "behaviors that undermine a culture of safety," to include:

» Corrective and disciplinary measures for those demonstrating the undermining behavior

» Protection for employees who report such behavior

» Response plans to help patients and their families who may witness undermining behavior

APPs must recognize the seriousness of disruptive behavior and use their leadership skills and wisdom to diffuse situations and responsibly report concerns to administration. The Joint Commission on Accreditation of Healthcare Organizations (2012) provides direction to all health care institutions that behaviors that undermine a culture of safety are not tolerated in the workplace.

Ineffective Leadership

The "ineffective leader" is a label that should not be quickly assigned, as there may be surrounding circumstances that interfere with a leader's progress. The journey of leaders holds periods when unexpected and external obstacles prevent success. A narrowed view by observers or team members that does not appreciate the leadership setting and accompanying situational challenges may inappropriately place blame on the leader. However, over time, the cause of any leadership concerns becomes clear. The leader who is unable to gain from mentoring or guidance, leading to persistent leadership quandaries, is considered an ineffective leader.

In these situations, the leader may resort to stepping back and devolving into an absent leader. If not, the leader will continue to create interference with forward progress due to ineffective actions, bringing more evidence to the cause of the concerns. Team members likely will eventually find voice to raise complaints. When done responsibly and with credible evidence, a registered complaint leads to decisions in restructuring the leadership. Opportunities to solve this type of dilemma with a clearly ineffective leader will only be delayed if the team members fail to respond.

The APP is in a position to understand the scope of the concerns about a leader and can navigate the situation to bring a productive discussion of how to regain effective leadership. The options may be difficult, including removal of the ineffective leader. That leader, however, is typically self-aware of the challenges and when this discussion maintains respect for all parties involved, the individual may be relieved to step away.

The APP should self-recognize her or his own ineffective leadership and let others assume the leadership role, respectful that the transition is best for the team. When possible, the APP may be of assistance in guiding a process of leadership transition that allows an ineffective leader to bow out and others, including the APP, to step up to carry leadership responsibilities.

Absent Leadership

A leadership position held by someone who is not showing any leadership results is demonstrating absent leadership. This is often a natural progression toward an end-stage of bad leadership if no other action has been successful in removing the leader. The leader is marginalized and limited in authority and responsibility, perhaps intentionally when the leadership role cannot be transitioned in other directions.

This may be a desirable path for a limited time, as the team finds alternative methods of functioning without the input and direction of the leader. However, it is taxing on the administrative and financial demands of the organization should there be a leader serving only as a placeholder for the position. Despite reprimand, an unethical, disruptive, or ineffective leader may continue to hold a leadership post but be unable to function. During a season of leadership transition, this may be necessary for a sequential organizational flow and progress.

Practical Analysis of Bad Leadership

When bad leadership occurs, exploring causative effects and classifying the type of leadership may offer direction for improving the leadership system. Of these five types of bad leadership described, some may require immediate attention (unethical), while others may respond to training and mentorship (incompetent), as summarized in Table 6.1.

The APP should give sufficient self-reflection to explore if he or she is a cause of the problem or is helping to solve the issues. When assured that the APP is external to the bad leadership, consider bringing together a balance of other key individuals who can help restore the leadership to an effective model.

THE DARK TRIAD

Over the past decade, study of employees and leaders who are toxic to the work environment have drawn the attention of researchers. These individuals are known to foster disharmony, favoritism, discord, and conflict. There is a bipolar continuum where each leader and team member is either working toward the team's success or working toward failure. Toxic leaders and team members are in the latter spectrum.

There are three traits surprisingly common in upper-level leadership roles across all types of organizations and work environments: narcissism, executive psychopathy, and Machiavellianism. Together, researchers have defined these as the "dark triad" (Paulhus & Williams, 2002). Any one of the three traits may be found among leaders at all levels, and all three traits hold intercorrelated effects (Jacobwitz & Egan, 2006).

Narcissism

The narcissist is prone to excessive self-admiration. While every person values being admired, when the individual is obsessed with self-interest it is an unhealthy condition of narcissism. At first glance, these individuals are often charming, engaging, and confident. Such characteristics are valued in leaders and lead to promotion to higher organizational levels. However, those working with the narcissist find the constant self-affirmation and egocentric worldview tiresome. Narcissists who are CEOs are prone to unethical behavior (Galperin, Bennett, & Aquino, 2010).

Executive Psychopathy

Psychopathy, a term popularized in the general press, is not a psychiatric diagnosis in the *Diagnostic and Statistical Manual of Mental Disorders* (*DSM*). Personality researchers, fiction authors, and criminal justice systems more commonly use the term. Researchers suggest in psychopathy that there is a disconnection between the brain and behavior, causing an absence of conscience (Richardson, 2000). It describes individuals who lack empathy and remorse, have difficulty maintaining interpersonal relationships, and are typically egocentric.

When an individual demonstrates this antisocial behavior in the workplace, *executive psychopathy* may apply (or other related terms such as "corporate psychopathy," "white-collar psychopathy," or "office psychopathy"). Executive psychopathic leaders are typically intelligent, sincere, and entertaining, but have shallow emotions. They are impatient, are unable to admit fault, and rely on temper tantrums and quickly blame others for mistakes. Masters at conning others, they praise those above while ridiculing others below. These individuals desire power and pursue the highest levels of leadership using deceit and sabotage.

Machiavellianism

Based on the short book, *The Prince*, Nicolò Machiavelli in the 1500s proposed a leadership style supporting behaviors that, regardless of being moral or amoral, were acceptable to achieve a worthwhile goal, including coercion, force, bribery, deceit, or worse, actions. The book remains a mainstay in the study of power and influence, warfare strategy, and politics. "Success at any cost" is the call of Machiavellianism applied to leadership. When leaders practice this in its subtlest forms (which are most effective and, therefore, most Machiavellian), these leaders achieve their goals. Their methods are secretive and manipulative, not easily recognized. With this duplicity, the leader is able to advance her or his goals without the full team being aware of the objectionable leadership strategies.

Early signs of Machiavellian leadership may be subtle compared to narcissistic or executive psychopathy. Questions should be raised when individual team members unexplainably lose commitment to the mission of the organization. Members close to the leader (in-group) who are not consumed by the leader's activities begin to withdraw. More distant team members (out-group) feel disenfranchised or are in disagreement with the leader's decisions and choose to withdraw.

Influence Tactics of the Dark Triad

The majority of individuals who exhibit the dark triad characteristics are nonviolent, and many have been able to use their disconnected, unwaveringly directed, and magnetic personalities to succeed in a variety of mainstream occupations.

Narcissists are recognized in using primarily *soft influence tactics* such as rational persuasion, inspirational appeal, and ingratiation (Jonason, Slomski, & Partyka, 2012), recognized as tactics with high or moderate effectiveness (see Chapter 2). Executive psychopaths are more likely to use direct coercion, coalition, or pressure (i.e., *hard influence tactics*). These latter tactics have lower effectiveness due to the more overt manipulation that is required. Machiavellianism was correlated with both soft and hard influence tactics.

In health care organizations, there are those across the team who occasionally exhibit elements of the dark triad without detracting from the success of the group. However, the toxic coworker or leader who routinely manifests such characteristics is likely discouraging team commitment, encouraging unethical behavior, and diminishing overall productivity.

The APP leader may miss seeing evidence of serious team problems due to the manipulative behaviors of the toxic member (see Case Study 1). In other situations, the APP leader may be too close to the situation to realize the effect on others or preoccupied and not vigilant enough to note concerns.

CASE STUDY 1

Jackson has been a physician assistant (PA) for over 10 years in an internal medicine group practice that serves primarily an adult population with multiple chronic conditions such as hypertension, diabetes, rheumatoid arthritis, and thyroid disease. He has oversight to a team of five other PAs and nurse practitioners (NPs) and was asked to meet with the group's CEO, Sandra, and the chief of their medical staff, Dr. Hutchins.

"Thanks for meeting with us on short notice," Sandra began. "We have some questions to ask you regarding one of our newer PAs, Quentin. Are you acquainted with him and his work?"

Jackson, caught off guard, answered, "Sure, I know of Quentin. He's been with us about 6 months now, seems punctual, and is a great team player. Everybody likes him so far. Is there a complaint against him?"

"That's what we're exploring, Jackson," Dr. Hutchins continued. "Have you seen anything that would concern you about his work?"

"Nothing I'm aware of," Jackson responded. "He's always positive when I'm around, and seems to have the respect of his nurses. Some patients already ask for him by name for appointments; I thought he was doing well. He participates in our monthly meeting and brings good questions to our journal club meetings. What have you heard?"

"We've asked one of the other PAs to come to you," Sandra said. "She's concerned that Quentin has falsified some information in the medical records of certain patients after he sees them. He apparently has documented that certain patients are to be scheduled with him on their return appointment."

"I see," Jackson nodded. "That's not how we do our patient follow-up. I'll be glad to mention that to him. I don't think he means anything by it."

Sandra continued, "And if that was all, we'd be fine with your plan. But there's more. Do you remember a patient last week whom Quentin was seeing? You apparently walked in on him during an exam while he was counting some pills in the patient's bottle."

"That's right. I needed to let him know that they needed him for surgery, so I just stepped in and gave him a quick reminder. When I opened the door, he was counting the patient's Vicodin, and I remember he accidentally dropped the bottle on the floor. A couple pills fell out of the bottle. I was going to help him pick them up but he just kicked them against the wall and said he would get them later. He said he didn't want the patient to take pills that had been on the floor. I know he remarked to the patient that he would be sure there was a refill to cover those pills. That all made sense to me."

"And did you see if he picked those pills off the floor?" Dr. Hutchins asked.

"No, I went to my next appointment," Jackson replied. "I told his nurse in the hall about what happened and she said she would get the pills when she cleaned the room."

"Yes, well, apparently when his nurse went in she didn't find any pills on the floor. When she asked Quentin, he reportedly said no pills spilled and all was fine."

"But I saw it," Jackson said. "He kicked the pills, pushed them with his shoe along the baseboard. I just thought he wanted them out of the way."

"That's what we heard," Dr. Hutchins responded. "Apparently he gave you something as a 'thank-you' that day?"

"Yes, that afternoon he sent me a bag of my favorite coffee beans." Jackson recalled. *"The note said something about how I was the best boss he'd ever had. Now I see what you're getting at."*

"Then yesterday," Sandra added, *"A nurse came to me lodging a harassment claim. I won't go into details, but there was enough there that I had to visit with Quentin right away. He denied it was true, said he was appalled that I would think he would stoop so low. Told me he thought we were both on the 'same team' and suggested I wasn't a very fair administrator. He said he thought that I knew him better than that."*

"So we came to you," Dr. Hutchins said, *"to see if you might have any insights to add. Have you had any concerns, or has Quentin done anything that might make you suspicious?"*

Situations such as Jackson is confronting are unfortunately too common. The APP leader must be alert to actions and attitudes among the health care team and be vigilant to pick up clues that suggest toxic behaviors.

CORRECTING TOXIC EMPLOYEES

When toxic employee behaviors are recognized, corrective action is required. Chapter 5 presents a method of corrective feedback to support a team member who is deficient in carrying out her or his responsibilities. When that feedback system is ineffective, the deficiencies in work performance persist, or toxic behaviors are documented, serious and formal intervention is required from the leadership to guide correction. APP leaders find themselves implementing this intervention with the goal of either correcting the behavior or facilitating the exit of the offensive party.

A leader without documented consultation with and support from the organization's administrative leadership should not initiate corrective action at this level. Human Resources personnel have expertise to guide the difficult steps in this process. The environment surrounding these issues can be volatile, and there are federal and state laws that protect employee rights. With the raised liability risk, it is imperative that the leader involved in the corrective action has guidance and support from the organization's administration.

With this documented support in place, the progressive steps of corrective action are verbal warning, written warning, suspension, and dismissal.

Verbal Warning

When more common measures of feedback and training have been ineffective, the first corrective action is a verbal warning. The leader at this point approaches the team member with the goal of yet improving the individual's work performance. A verbal warning does not hold an expectation that the team member's employment is at risk of termination. The focus is on addressing the undesired behavior with clear requirements that should correct the behavior.

To demonstrate the leader's support of the team member, a clear plan including required actions by the team member is needed. The plan may address behaviors to be avoided with actions that carry a more positive message of "do this," rather than only a series of "don't do that" steps. Suggestions for these positive actions that may apply in certain situations include asking the team member to:

» Initiate meeting with anyone who holds misperceptions to allay any resentment and reaffirm the commitment to being a willing and positive member of the team

» Apologize to those who have been on the receiving end of any unprofessional behavior or been otherwise offended

» Personally demonstrate a commitment to trust in and support of the leader (e.g., leadership buy-in at 70%–80%)

» Encourage and facilitate the achievement of other team members

The leader should plan to meet routinely with the team member over a limited time period to keep communication open and build up the professional relationship (e.g., a 30-minute, weekly meeting for 4 to 6 weeks). If that is not possible, establish a clear point of follow-up, such as meeting in 2 weeks, so that the team member can provide a progress update. That time allows for discussion of any challenges; the leader can encourage the team member over indications of progress and the relationship is further strengthened.

The leader must clearly communicate that this conversation is a "verbal warning" and document a report of this exchange, including the plan for improvement, in the team member's employment record. Provide the verbal warning report to the team member with a request that receipt of the report be acknowledged.

Written Warning

The stakes are raised with a written warning, indicating that the standard of improvement expected after the verbal warning was not achieved. This should involve another conversation, with an actual hard copy document of written warning included as a part of the conversation or immediately sent following this new verbal exchange. The tone of the conversation and written warning still supports the individual to become a valuable, productive team member. The discussion builds on earlier conversations but must reinforce the expected performance of the team member within an explicit timeframe. The written warning should give detail to these expectations and include reference to potential outcomes if the performance goals are not reached, such as taking disciplinary action. The team member should acknowledge receipt and understanding of the written warning by a return signature.

Suspension

If performance goals of the team member are not reached within the established timeframe in the written warning, the next step is to suspend the individual from work without pay for a limited time period. This suspension is a disciplinary action managed with direction from the organization's administrative leadership (e.g., human resources or department management). The team member should use the time to reflect on and determine his or her commitment to the team. Upon return, the leader should expect that the individual has resolved whatever issues were preventing the attainment of the performance goals. The team member may elect to separate from the organization if disagreements persist, which may at this point be the best outcome for all those involved.

Dismissal

This action occurs after the verbal and written warnings and the suspension as the final act terminating employment and the team's relationship with the individual. Despite concerted efforts to help the individual reach the performance expectations and resolve barriers, the goals were not reached. As a last resort, the administrative leadership, based on recommendations including those from the APP leader, has no recourse but to dismiss the individual, allowing both parties to head in separate directions.

BAD LEADERSHIP PREVENTION

Bad leadership, at its core, is a failure of communication. The source of the poor communication may be problematic with complicated root causes at play, but the action that has failed is communication. Therefore, the key to avoiding bad leadership is effective communication, emphasizing two elements: speaking and listening.

A study at Columbia University's Business School explored speaking and listening abilities in 274 MBA students (36% women, mean age 28.3) and found that of these two, listening well proved to be the more influential trait (Ames, Maissen, & Brockner, 2012). This is contrary to what many tout as a strength of most leaders. Leadership education (including this text) emphasizes the need to cast vision, convey a clear sense of direction, and use compelling language to persuade others. From this study, speaking well combined with listening well brings the higher ratings for being influential.

EFFECTIVE LISTENING

Listening well takes time, but it is not as simple as giving others around the leader the occasion to speak themselves. *Active listening* involves listening skills to help others open up and elaborate on what they are saying. Team members who find their leader is a good listener feel that they are heard *and understood*. They respect the leader for being open to discuss alternative or opposing ideas. The leader who is skilled at active listening will have greater influence.

Elements of Active Listening

CONSCIOUSLY PRESENT
In the busy and often hectic life of the APP, the idea of being consciously present can be challenging. Effective listening is impaired when the leader is distracted, preoccupied, or otherwise unable to intently listen in the moment. Introduced in Chapter 3, the practice of mindfulness can be helpful to being consciously present. Three habits to avoid in active listening include mind-wandering, multitasking, and thinking ahead (Goh, 2012).

» **Mind-wandering:** Mental clutter causes thinking to dart back and forth between the topic at hand and other issues requiring attention. The APP needs to control the focus of the mind to stay at the task of fully listening in the present to the person talking.

» **Multitasking:** APPs may be tempted to finish an email while someone is speaking, or check cell phone messages, take notes (mental or otherwise), or complete other tasks while in conversation. To listen actively, the APP must set aside all tasks and responsibilities to focus on this discussion.

» **Thinking ahead:** Sometimes leaders are in one of two modes, talking or waiting to talk. Rather than mentally planning what needs to be said next, the APP should avoid this urge and stay reflective on what is being heard in the present. Consciously digesting what the other person says needs to be intentional and obvious, perhaps even stating, "I want to think about that before I respond."

Without extra effort, the listener naturally holds mental screens so that what is heard passes through the listener's own agenda, fears, and judgment, leading to selectively "hearing what you want to hear." The active listener strains to listen fully, paying attention without distraction, using nonverbal displays (described further), and clearly making space for the other person to express opinions.

PHYSICALLY PRESENT

In addition to being consciously present, active listening involves being physically present in the moment, as measured by body posture. Utilizing these physical indications of actively listening such as leaning forward, tilting the head in interest and head nodding to encourage the listener are powerful in communicating to the speaker that the APP is fully listening. Chief among these are maintaining eye contact; holding the speaker's gaze communicates respect and understanding. Misunderstandings and antagonistic language are often avoided when the APP is able to look directly into the eyes of the team member.

RESIST SPEAKING

It requires discipline, but the practice of pausing after the other person finishes speaking conveys active listening. Interrupting, even to agree, does not allow the speaker to be fully heard. Avoid making jokes in response to what the other person says, as it can be distracting and interpreted as diminishing the importance of what was said. Finishing the other person's sentence does not allow the speaker to personally share his or her own thinking.

CONVEY TRUST

Marketing and sales strategies have taught that there is a direct correlation between effective listening and trust. Telling of the times, members of Congress rank lowest on perceived honesty in the annual Gallup poll that asks Americans to rank 22 professions on honesty and ethical standards. Car salespeople rank next to the lowest, both professions recognized for talking much and listening little. On the top of the poll: nurses, pharmacists, and physicians (Norman, 2016). Nurses have secured the number-one ranking every year since 2001. The marker most indicative that nurses can be trusted is the confident belief that they listen to and understand their patients.

APPs who actively listen use the same skills as applied to establishing patient rapport and taking a medical history (e.g., asking open-ended questions, clarifying and summarizing what was said, and validating the patient's feelings). These communication skills translate well in any discussion to actively listen and convey trust.

EMPATHIC UNDERSTANDING

Active listening shows empathy by body language and responses. People recognize they are heard when the listener identifies with the emotions behind what is shared. Empathic understanding offers a response to the individual's emotions. When conversations are difficult, the APP should express a full understanding of what is heard by offering empathic responses that show care and support.

A study at Mayo Clinic Arizona followed health care providers who participated in a 1-day course on communication skills focused on the PEARLS approach to active listening and relationship building (see Table 6.2 for a description of PEARLS). Their results from 80 providers evaluated by over 3,500 patient surveys compared patient satisfaction outcomes 1 year before and 1 year after course participation (Kennedy, Fasolino, & Gullen, 2014). Statistically significant improvements were noted in listening, knowing the patient as a person, and overall quality of care, among others. The APP who seeks to improve listening skills may find the PEARLS approach useful.

TABLE 6.2 PEARLS Relationship-Building Statements

Empathic Category	Sample Empathic Statement
Partnership	I really want to work on this with you
	I bet we can figure this out together
Empathy	I can feel your enthusiasm as you talk
	I can hear your concern
Acknowledgment	You clearly put a lot of work into this
	You invested in this, and it shows
Respect	I've always appreciated your creativity
	There's no doubt you know a lot about this
Legitimation	This would be hard for anyone
	Who wouldn't be worried about something like this?
Support	I'd like to help you with this
	I want to see you succeed

Source: From "How thinking like a hostage negotiator can make you more persuasive, influential, and motivating" from Friedman, R. (2014). *The best place to work: The art and science of creating an extraordinary workplace.* copyright © 2014 by Ron Friedman. Used by permission of Berkley, an imprint of Penguin Publishing Group, a division of Penguin Random House LLC. All rights reserved.

Combining Effective Speaking and Listening

The effective APP leader is able to persuade others to change their opinions and build coalitions to get things done. These reflect effective speaking skills highlighted by compelling logic and vivid images. Leader communication that is clear, concise, to the point, and brief is exemplary. The APP's communication skills are enhanced by strong listening skills. The APP who is also able to help others volunteer their thoughts and who listens effectively to criticism and alternative points of view will avoid the pitfalls of bad leaders.

EXERCISE 6.1 ACTIVE LISTENING EXERCISE

This exercise can be completed in less than 10 minutes and can be done in groups of two in a small group, staff meeting, or classroom.

1. *Self-select a partner with whom to work. Determine who will first be the "speaker" and who will be the "listener."*

2. *The speaker tells the listener a story about the most exciting vacation experienced (or other highlight from lived life). The listener should demonstrate the opposite of active listening (e.g., be distracted by technology, interrupt, avoid eye contact, and generally not listen well).*

3. *After about 2 minutes, halt the story and discuss perceptions and feelings within each pair.*

4. *Switch the roles of "speaker" and "listener" in the same pair.*

5. *The new speaker now reports on what happened yesterday, beginning with her or his usual morning routine. The new listener employs active listening skills (e.g., asking questions for clarification, using verbal and nonverbal cues to show interest, maintaining eye contact, avoiding all distractions, and generally being fully present).*

6. *After another 2 minutes, halt the story and have the pair discuss new perceptions and feelings.*

The applications from this exercise, adding value to the benefits of active listening, will be self-evident and highlighted in a group time of sharing.

SUMMARY POINTS

1. An APP in health environments does not have to look far to find examples of bad leadership. While the leader may be struggling due to external and uncontrollable circumstances, in other situations the right person is not leading. The APP should learn to be self-aware of his or her leadership effectiveness, as well as be vigilant in identifying other leaders who are struggling. After identifying the cause of the weakened leadership, classifying the bad leadership into one of the following categories will offer a direction for solving the concerns: unethical, incompetent, ineffective, disruptive, ineffective, or absent leadership. Bad leadership can stem from personality or behavioral traits that are summarized as the "dark triad": narcissism, executive psychopathy, and Machiavellianism. When leaders routinely manifest these traits, a toxic leader exists and likely needs displacement.

2. When the APP has oversight of or influence over an individual who is not contributing to the success of the team, corrective action is indicated. If given authority, the APP leader should take the responsibility to engage the team member in support of improved work performance. If casual interactions and counsel are not fruitful, a more formal process is indicated. With the support of upper-level management, the APP may be in a position to initiate a verbal warning, followed by a written warning if improvement is not achieved. Following the organization's protocols and human resources guidance, the team member may require suspension for a limited time if the goals of work performance are not met. The final step in this formal process is termination.

3. The best practice the APP can maintain to avoid bad leadership pitfalls is to communicate well and particularly to listen well. The art of active listening includes specific elements: being consciously present, being physically present, resisting the urge to speak, conveying trust, and showing empathic understanding. These aspects of active listening require attention and focus, and APPs should regularly exercise their listening skills.

REFERENCES

Ames, D., Maissen, L. B., & Brockner, J. (2012). The role of listening in interpersonal influence. *Journal of Research in Personality, 26*(3), 345–349.

Friedman, R. (2014). *The best place to work: The art and science of creating an extraordinary workplace* (pp. 177–198). New York, NY: Perigee.

Galperin, B. L., Bennett, R. J., & Aquino, K. (2010). Status differentiation and the protean self: A social-cognitive model of unethical behavior in organizations. *Journal of Business Ethics, 98*, 407–424.

Goh, E. C. L. (2012). Integrating mindfulness and reflection in the teaching and learning of listening skills for undergraduate social work students in Singapore. *Social Work Education, 31*(5), 587–604.

Jacobwitz, S., & Egan, V. (2006). The dark triad and normal personality traits. *Personality and Individual Differences, 40*, 331–339.

Joint Commission on Accreditation of Healthcare Organizations. (2012). Leadership standard clarified to address behaviors that undermine a safety culture. *Joint Commission Perspectives, 32*(1), 7.

Jonason, P. K., Slomski, S., & Partyka, J. (2012). The dark triad at work: How toxic employees get their way. *Personality and Individual Differences, 52*, 449–453.

Kennedy, D. M., Fasolino, F. P., & Gullen, D. J. (2014). Improving patient experiences through provider communication skills building. *Patient Experience Journal, 1*(1), 56–60.

Norman, J. (2016). Americans rate healthcare providers high on honesty, ethics. *Gallup.* Retrieved from http://www.gallup.com/poll/200057/americans-rate -healthcare-providers-high-honesty-ethics.aspx?version=print

Paulhus, D. L., & Williams, K. M. (2002). The dark triad of personality: Narcissism, Machiavellianism and psychopathy. *Journal of Research in Personality, 36*, 556–563.

Richardson, D. J. (2000). Affective style, psychopathology, and resilience: Brain mechanisms and plasticity. *American Psychologist, 55*(11), 1196–1214.

Rosenstein, A., & O'Daniel, M. (2008). Invited article: Managing disruptive physician behavior: Impact on staff relationships and patient care. *Neurology, 70*(17), 1564–1570.

PART 2
Administrative Leadership Strategies for PAs and NPs

7
FINANCIAL PRINCIPLES IN CLINICAL LEADERSHIP

CRITICAL THINKING QUESTIONS

» **What principles of financial management are common in cost-effective health care organizations?**

» **What measures are useful to advanced practice provider (APP) leaders to determine productivity outcomes with fiscal responsibility?**

» **How does the APP leader contribute to the financial leadership of a health care system?**

Health care systems cannot exist and grow without covering the expenses of providing the care. The role of the APP leader includes the fiscal responsibility to maintain affordable health care and derive an income to meet the expenses of care. The business of health care requires generating revenue to invest in the health care system, support the high quality of care provided, and advance services to meet the needs of those served.

The APP serves as one part of a complex supply chain to deliver health care. Because of the comprehensive care the typical APP provides, a perspective of health care delivery may be confined to what occurs between the APP and the patient (see Figure 7.1A). However, even in the caring for a straightforward health need (e.g., a complaint of a sore throat or an ankle sprain), there are other necessary components of the health care system beyond the limited APP-to-patient description (see Figure 7.1B). The resources tapped by the APP to provide the care needed broadens this network to include services supporting the clinical evaluation and therapeutic modalities of medications and interventional therapies.

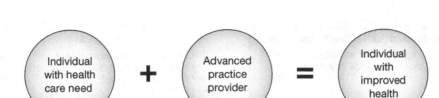

FIGURE 7.1A Basic perception of health care delivery between APP and patient.
APP, advanced practice provider.

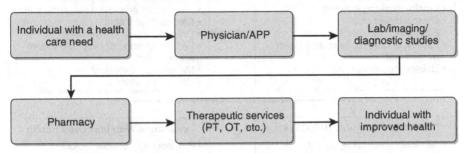

FIGURE 7.1B Basic perception of health care delivery between health care system and patient.
APP, advanced practice provider; OT, occupational therapy; PT, physical therapy.

Even in this simple patient care episode, the costs associated with the system of care are multiple. At each step of care, there are support services behind the clinician or other provider (i.e., lab, imaging, or other diagnostic technologist; pharmacist; other therapeutic provider, etc.). Each component involves administrative support, clerical and billing services, overhead and facility upkeep, and liability insurance coverage (see Figure 7.1C). Depending on the services provided, there are additional nursing and clinical staff support, equipment maintenance, product storage, and inventory needs. Other costs will vary depending on the local needs and services of the local provider. For example, some of these services depend on advertising to draw a customer base.

This single patient care visit multiplied represents all patient encounters, broadly expanded to cover varying health care needs. Additional factors with financial implications include procuring material supplies, adjusting to varying patient volume and employee workloads, staying relevant to health care technology and advancements, conforming to regulatory requirements, and meeting consumer satisfaction needs.

Place this health care delivery model into an inpatient care system, a residential care system, an emergency room, a surgical suite, and alternative

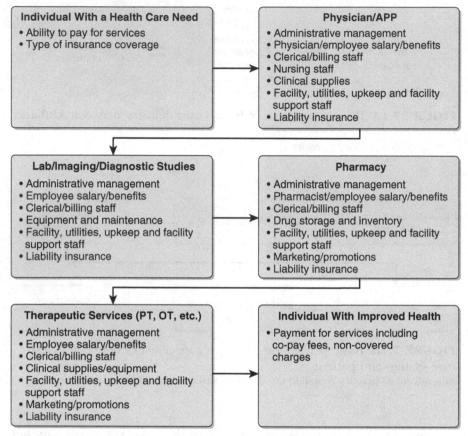

Individual With a Health Care Need
- Ability to pay for services
- Type of insurance coverage

Physician/APP
- Administrative management
- Physician/employee salary/benefits
- Clerical/billing staff
- Nursing staff
- Clinical supplies
- Facility, utilities, upkeep and facility support staff
- Liability insurance

Lab/Imaging/Diagnostic Studies
- Administrative management
- Employee salary/benefits
- Clerical/billing staff
- Equipment and maintenance
- Facility, utilities, upkeep and facility support staff
- Liability insurance

Pharmacy
- Administrative management
- Pharmacist/employee salary/benefits
- Clerical/billing staff
- Drug storage and inventory
- Facility, utilities, upkeep and facility support staff
- Marketing/promotions
- Liability insurance

Therapeutic Services (PT, OT, etc.)
- Administrative management
- Employee salary/benefits
- Clerical/billing staff
- Clinical supplies/equipment
- Facility, utilities, upkeep and facility support staff
- Marketing/promotions
- Liability insurance

Individual With Improved Health
- Payment for services including co-pay fees, non-covered charges

FIGURE 7.1C Examples of economic costs from Figure 7.1B in basic perception of health care delivery between health care system and patient.
APP, advanced practice provider; OT, occupational therapy; PT, physical therapy.

health care systems and the economic implications become increasingly complex requiring careful management. The APP leader is a steward over one or more of the components of these systems, responsible for conserving the expense of care while providing for the advancement of quality.

CASE STUDY 1

Chelsea is a family nurse practitioner who has been staffing the urgent care clinic at a drugstore chain in her community for 8 years. She has grown from managing this clinic to now overseeing two other retail-based clinics in town and four clinics in each of four neighboring communities. The clinics are open for at least 4 to 6 hours each day, varying from morning, afternoon, and evening shifts. Chelsea sees patients during three shifts each week, and the rest of her full-time work involves supporting nearly 20 nurse practitioners (NPs) and physician assistants (PAs), training providers and coordinating services at all seven clinics. Each clinic has limited lab facilities, typically providing only strept screening, automated urinalysis, and blood glucose testing. Chelsea helps maintain consulting and referral relationships at family medicine clinics in each community. Lab and x-ray services, linked to each clinic through independent providers, require unique fees.

The regional chief financial officer (CFO) of the drugstore asked to meet with Chelsea this week. He provided a review of data collected over the past 3 years of the clinics' services. The good news was that patient volume and revenue exceeded projections. Patient satisfaction scores were generally strong. The bad news was that utilization of the ancillary lab and x-ray services had increased, creating additional charges through the clinic that resulted in less-than-expected net income for the clinics. The CFO presented even more difficult news: Data from the company's clinics in neighboring states show that clinics staffed by physicians did not utilize ancillary services as often for the same diagnoses as the clinics under Chelsea's direction. The measure evaluated utilization of lab and x-ray for diagnoses of acute pharyngitis, acute bronchitis, ankle sprain, and urinary tract infection. The data suggested that the APPs were ordering too many lab tests and x-rays compared to the physician-staffed clinics for those diagnoses.

Chelsea was to explore this information with her staff of APPs and prepare a proposal to meet new revenue projections for the next year. The CFO gave her the following options to help meet these budget expectations:

- *Reduce utilization of lab and x-ray services by 20%*

- *Increase general patient volume that does not require ancillary services by 15%*

- *Eliminate one full-time APP and hire part-time APPs to cover the schedule, reducing the expense of full-time benefits*

- *Decrease the 4% salary/wages increase previously planned for the next year*

Other cost-saving measures such as reducing clinical and office supplies or curtailing custodial services were welcome, but would not likely be sufficient to meet the projected budget shortfall without adopting at least one of the other recommendations.

The CFO gave Chelsea 2 weeks to meet with her staff and recommend what measures should be taken.

BUDGETS, CASH FLOW, AND OPERATING MARGINS

In Case Study 1, the CFO for the drugstore chain maintains a system that tracks expenses and income to establish a budget for the financial outcomes expected for the clinics Chelsea manages. There are different styles of budgeting, and in Case Study 1A, she learns the budgeting style of her employer. It is beneficial to know the overall budget philosophy of the institution; it can be generally classified as some blend of centralized and decentralized budgeting.

Centralized Versus Decentralized Budgeting

A centralized budget keeps all budget decisions with a central administrator. Small organizations or a solo practice clinic may function well by a centralized budget. Because of multifaceted departments and services that have unique cost and revenue streams, most health care systems work within a combination of some aspects of both centralized and decentralized budgeting. For example, a high-level administrator has oversight to certain budget areas (centralized budget) with local departments or service areas within the system managing their own budgets (decentralized budget). Those areas with decentralized budgeting report their department budget to the central office monthly or quarterly to maintain accountability, but generally maintain responsibility to manage their own department's expenses and income.

When financial circumstances are difficult, centralized budgeting offers a prudent way to steer the organization through the challenges, leaving the tough decisions to the highest level of administration. Central budgeting may also be effective for departments that have no clear performance indicators but provide basic services required for the organization (e.g., a budget for standard equipment, computers, and printers). By a centralized budget, the costs can remain uniform and controlled across the organization but maintained to ensure the services are functional.

Decentralized budgeting is more appropriate for local departments that have clear performance measures. This also can offer an element of healthy competition between departments as a motivation to be cost-effective while maintaining high-quality services and high patient satisfaction.

In Case Study 1, Chelsea is working within a decentralized budgeting system; she has local control for determining the expenses. The company has central oversight of the budget, setting performance standards. This would represent a mix of centralized and decentralized budgeting.

After distinguishing the balance of centralized and decentralized budgeting, a line-item budget specifies by a spreadsheet (ledger) the individual categories of revenue and cost in single lines. From that spreadsheet, the plan for managing revenue and costs are developed by different types of budget approaches, such as zero-based budgeting, incremental budgeting, program budgeting, performance-based budgeting, or responsibility-centered budgeting.

ZERO-BASED BUDGETING

At the beginning of every budget planning period, *zero-based budgeting* requires that the previous year's budget be cleared (at "zero") for every department. Then every department requests funding with appropriate justification. This method controls unnecessary costs since requested funds are allocated for a specific purpose, limiting waste and discretionary spending. The planning period is more time-consuming under this budgeting style and may be more stringent than necessary for some organizations.

INCREMENTAL BUDGETING

This traditional budget model uses previous budgets to base funding levels for the new budget period. Budget increases or reductions (by increments up or down) are determined from the outcomes of the historical budget and implemented uniformly across the organization. If the organization has predictable and stable trends for expected costs and revenues, *incremental budgeting* is an effective model and not as demanding to prepare and implement. However, in times of economic stress requiring frequent and complex change, such as today's health care environment, this model limits the ability to respond quickly to insurance and regulatory changes.

PROGRAM BUDGETING

By a mixed centralized and decentralized budgeting process, *program budgeting* allocates funding to programs that have the greatest needs or greatest opportunities for financial gain. Individual programs make budget proposals and central administrators determine tailored allocations for each program. Programs function within the allocated budget with more freedom to make adjustments fitting their local needs and opportunities. This method can be troublesome because central administrators make decisions affecting individual programs based on projections that may not be realized. Competition between programs is common, which can be positive or negative depending on the organizational culture.

PERFORMANCE-BASED BUDGETING

Whereas program budgeting allocates funds based on the projections of income or other beneficial gains of individual programs, *performance-based budgeting* allocates funds based on past performance using defined outcomes measures. As health care systems find revenue streams based on pay-for-performance-type measures, those organizations may adopt budgeting measures to increase those revenue streams. The planning period must include a review of performance measures (requiring prior data collection and analysis) to measure outcomes. In Case Study 1, Chelsea is working for a company with performance-based budgeting.

RESPONSIBILITY-CENTERED BUDGETING

Responsibility-centered budgeting reflects a larger management philosophy. The budget follows the mission of the organization, with funds allocated to support the achievement of priorities related to the mission. Typically, those areas served by the organization's mission also generate the highest income, so this model may be similar to performance-based budgeting. However, some organizational missions in health care may serve populations that do not offer a high revenue stream (particularly vulnerable or underserved populations). The mission gives priority to funding those programs separate from economic outcomes. When governmental funding or private contributions are available, responsibility-centered budgeting functions effectively as those funds are distinctly available apart from funds generated directly by payment for services. Responsibility-based budgeting puts departments or programs at risk for cuts if they are not supported by mission and do not generate income.

Cash Flow

Regardless of the type of health care organization budgeting, bills for patient care services are often paid by installments over time by insurance agencies or patients. Organizational costs for technology, clinical research, facility expansion, recruiting experts, and medical enhancements are funded through multiyear expense lines. While a well-framed budget will account for the staggered payment of costs and generation of revenue over time, charges will still require cash payments. Cash flow represents the real dollars exchanged as revenue comes in or cost payments go out. Sources of revenue include payment for services (accounts receivable), investment income, capital contributions, and sale of assets. The outflow of cash goes to wages and salaries, payments for supplies, purchases of equipment, facility needs, and investment contributions. In uncertain times, cash balances are increased to maintain cash flow or credit is secured to advance the organization.

Operating Margin

The operating margin is calculated from any type of budget to determine the profit ratio. This is the proportion of profit from the income generated after expenses are paid. The calculation subtracts total expenses from total income, deriving the operating income. Dividing the operating income by the original total income is equal to the operating margin.

$$\frac{(\text{Total income} - \text{Total expenses})}{\text{Total income}} = \frac{\text{Operating income}}{\text{Total income}} = \text{Operating margin}$$

In an organization that has a monthly income of $800,000 and total expenses for the month of $650,000, the operating margin is 18.75% as shown using this following formula:

$$\frac{(\$800K - \$650K)}{\$800K} = \frac{\$150K}{\$800K} = 18.75\% = \text{Operating margin}$$

The target for a desired operating margin varies greatly between organizations. The higher the operating margin, the better the financial position as interpreted by the owners, investors, and long-term lenders.

REVENUE SYSTEMS

A budget is useless without some expectation of income. Determining the source and stability of the revenue stream is necessary. There may be other sources of income from investments, foundation resources, grants and governmental programs, but reimbursement for health care services is the main source of revenue for most health care systems. Third-party payers cover these costs, identified as insurance agencies that are under contract by the "second-party" (often the government or employers) to pay for services provided to the "first party" (the patient).

Historical Perspective

Prior to the 1930s in the United States, individuals paid directly for their health care, often in cash, produce, or exchange of services. During the era of the Great Depression, the American Hospital Association developed a program allowing individuals to pay a monthly fee (premium) to purchase insurance covering hospital charges when and if needed. The program, called *Blue Cross*, was so successful that the American Medical Association began a similar program for individuals to purchase insurance to cover physicians' charges, called *Blue Shield*. These programs were prosperous and grew into the major third-party payer of today, joined by many other commercial health insurance programs.

The U.S. government instituted Medicare in the 1960s to support the health care needs of the elderly. Medicare Part A was a compulsory insurance to help cover hospital charges for the elderly. Provided at no cost and funded by taxes on each American taxpayer's employment income, the program remains available to the nation's elders when they leave the workforce. Medicare Part B similarly provides reimbursement for physician services, though individuals participating in Part B are required to pay a small monthly premium payment. State Medicaid programs are developed with costs shared by federal and state governments to provide reimbursement for the health care services provided to families in poverty. Today, those receiving Medicare or Medicaid pay a portion of their health care charges, but the governmental third-party payers cover approximately 75% to 85% of the health care costs for these populations.

These programs help control costs and distribute the burden of health care expenses. There has been no system proven to fit well, and long-term sustainability of these systems remains in question. Various methods have been developed to manage reimbursement, such as pay-for-service, diagnosis-related groups, global payments, and relative value units, among others.

Pay for Service

Sometimes referred to as cost-based reimbursement, this is a traditional payment system where the payer (often a governmental or insurance agency) and provider negotiate payment for services. It may be *retrospective*, with payment occurring after services are rendered, or *prospective*, with payment made prior to the actual services based on a projected expense. In prospective payment, if the predetermined amount is exceeded (e.g., the patient has complications or other health issues arise that need attention requiring additional expense), the payer may not be obligated to pay additional costs.

Diagnosis-Related Groups

For inpatient care, Medicare patients can be categorized by their diagnosis with an established fee determined for each diagnosis-related group (DRG). Reimbursement rates are set based on a review of national data tracking typical care and related expenses by diagnosis. Other commercial insurance companies have adopted the Medicare DRG fee schedule. Hospitals are expected to find that, on average, their costs will be covered by the DRG fee structure, as some patients will fare better than the national average and other patients will fare worse. By this method, hospitals share in the costs associated with patients suffering complications and extended hospital stays. However, some health care institutions have been prone to discharge patients earlier than desired to stay under the DRG reimbursement value, bringing a margin of profit at the risk of lowering the quality of care. DRG payment methods remain the principal means of reimbursing hospitals for acute inpatient care in most high-income countries and are being implemented in low- and middle-income countries (Mathauer & Wittenbecher, 2013).

Global Payment

Institutions may receive routine fixed payment for services that generally meet expected costs, maintaining a stable revenue stream. On a quarterly or annual basis, the payer reviews the actual services recorded and makes a one-time adjustment to meet the actual expenses over that period. Sometimes referred to as "bundled payments," the fixed payment includes a variety of services based on estimates of predicted usage.

Relative Value Units

The means to receive payment for the clinical services of the provider is associated with set fees, more often now determined by a calculation of the work relative value unit (wRVU). This method of compensation for physician and APP services is determined by productivity factors that are adjusted based on geographic location and external factors such as malpractice costs and costs associated with the specialty practice setting.

The calculation used to determine the wRVU varies. For example, Medicare uses a formula developed by the American Medical Association (AMA) Specialty Society Relative Value Scale Update Committee (RUC), and then adds its own conversion factor to the final fee. For specific procedures, there are defined relative value units (RVUs) based on the procedural code it is assigned in the Current Procedural Terminology (CPT) manual, also published by the AMA.

The system of RVUs can unfairly hide the actual productivity of the APP. In global (or bundled) payments in a surgical practice, the preoperative and postsurgical care provided by the APP is notable, but those duties are assigned an RVU of 0 because all aspects of the surgical care and operative procedures are combined in one global payment. This does not recognize the productivity of the surgical APP (Pickard, 2014). Similarly, there are wRVU calculations utilized only for physician services, and the APP associated with the practice does not gain a unique accounting of productivity if the services rendered are filed under the physician's wRVU.

Newer wRVU methods are providing a better record of the specific productivity of each health care provider. APPs should understand the wRVU method used in their respective clinical practices to ensure an accurate accounting of their work.

MACRA AND THE QUALITY PAYMENT PROGRAM

The Medicare Access and CHIP (Child's Health Insurance Program) Re-authorization Act (MACRA) is U.S. federal legislation passed and signed into law in 2015 that brought several quality reporting and reimbursement programs into one: the Quality Payment Program (QPP).

As the transition year, 2017 brings important reimbursement advantages to all health professionals, including APPs. The QPP includes several different incentive payment programs for reporting certain clinical services, titled by the acronyms MIPS and Advanced APMs (see following sections). With a few exceptions, the Centers for Medicare and Medicaid Services (CMS) requires APPs to participate in at least one type of these programs if providing care to individuals with Medicare.

Merit-Based Incentive Payments System

APPs can elect to participate in one or more projects created within the Merit-based Incentive Payments System (MIPS). These projects provide payment incentives based on evidence-based and practice-specific measures of high-quality care as reported by patient outcome data or documentation of quality improvement activities. Examples of merit-based practice activities include meeting established benchmarks for the following patient conditions, among many others:

- » Use of topical rather than systemic therapies for acute otitis externa
- » Management of blood pressure in adult kidney disease
- » Appropriate antibiotic usage for adult sinusitis
- » Appropriate antiplatelet therapy for coronary artery disease
- » Optimal asthma control

MIPS also includes quality improvement activities in the local practice setting, such as:

- » Surveying the patient safety culture in the local practice
- » Registration in the national Prescription Drug Monitoring Program
- » Utilization of depression-screening tools
- » Patient screening and brief counseling for unhealthy alcohol use

Advanced Alternative Payment Models

Alternative payment models (APMs) offer payment incentives for cost-effective and high-quality care. Advanced APMs increase the payment incentives in return for the practice assuming a greater risk of the patients' outcomes. For example, one advanced APM is a partnership between clinicians and the CMS to explore and evaluate new ways to improve care for patients with end-stage renal disease. Another example evaluates the care provided to Medicare patients requiring hip or knee replacement surgery.

Improvement in the quality of patient care is the goal of the QPP by creating incentives for health care providers, including APPs. Compared to past models that are volume driven (revenue increased by a greater volume of patients and services provided), QPP motivates clinical practices to pursue value. CMS pledges to support rural practices by providing technical support for establishing MIPS activities. It behooves all APPs to explore what activities are best suited in their local practice to gain these incentives.

CASE STUDY 1 (CONTINUED)

Chelsea met with her fellow APPs to discuss the CFO's report and the options of how to reduce the ancillary charges or increase the clinic's revenue. They reviewed the 3-year data showing the high patient volume, overall revenue, and positive patient satisfaction scores. They could not find fault with the data behind the increased utilization of lab and x-ray. While surprised, they had to agree with the comparison figures from other physician-staffed clinics that from the four diagnoses used in the performance measures (acute pharyngitis, acute bronchitis, ankle sprain, and urinary tract infections), the APPs as a group ordered more ancillary tests.

Chelsea led the group through a discussion of the options presented by the CFO with the following summaries of advantages and disadvantages:

- *Reduce utilization of lab and x-ray services by 20%*

  - *Advantages: Directly solves the budget needs.*

  - *Disadvantages: Limits the diagnostic tools the APPs have found helpful; may diminish the accuracy of diagnostic decisions, diminishing the quality of patient care.*

- *Increase general patient volume not requiring ancillary services by 15%*

  - *Advantages: Directly solves the budget needs.*

  - *Disadvantages: Requires untested marketing strategies with an uncertain effect on clinic reputation and patient appeal. Targeting populations by specific diagnoses that do not require ancillary services is untenable.*

- *Eliminate one full-time APP and hire part-time APPs to cover the schedule, reducing the expense of full-time benefits*

  - *Advantages: Limits the effect of budget constraints to one person losing full-time employment and benefits.*

  - *Disadvantages: No current employee is willing to transition to part-time, and the loss of anyone from the current team is undesirable.*

- *Decrease the planned 4% salary/wages increase*

  - *Advantages: No APP loses employment.*

  - *Disadvantages: Current APP salaries are under national and local norms so some APPs may seek other positions if salaries do not keep pace with the market. This brings a low morale among the APP staff as the customer satisfaction scores indicated they were exceeding expectations, yet they would miss fair compensation for their work.*

Chelsea challenged her team during the meeting with determining what recommendations they should make to the CFO.

COMPLEXITY OF REVENUE MANAGEMENT

The cluster of acronyms associated with the MACRA legislation (i.e., CMS, QPP, MIPS, and APMs) is evidence that the pattern of revenue paths is complicated and confusing. In Case Study 1, Chelsea is required to navigate decentralized budgeting, performance-based budgeting, wRVUs, and various revenue streams to help protect the employment of her fellow APPs. More importantly, the decisions she makes will affect the quality of care her practice setting delivers. However, resources are available by sponsoring governmental agencies, professional organizations, and local health care experts, easily accessed by the Internet or local contacts.

Productivity Comparisons

Comparisons between health care organizations or local delivery systems need to consider a variety of influences that affect productivity outcomes. Different practice settings, geographical locations, clinical services, and professional staffing all contribute to the dynamics of health care delivery. External market forces such as the local economy, availability of other services, and the health culture of the community are among many factors that influence productivity.

A recent study of NPs and PAs in the Veterans Health Administration (VHA) assessed clinical productivity (Moran et al., 2016). The researchers used each clinician's wRVU divided by the direct clinical full-time equivalent (FTE) for the individual (1.0 FTE was equal to at least 35 hours per week). While their clinical services were all within the same organization, a number of factors correlated with APP productivity. The wRVUs were measured over the 2014 fiscal year for nearly 6,000 APPs (70% NPs and 30% PAs). APPs in rural areas were more productive compared to their nonrural counterparts (NPs 7% more productive, PAs 15% more productive). Those in nonteaching hospitals were also more productive (NPs 11% more productive, PAs 8% more productive). APPs in VHA primary care were 9% (NP) and 17% (PA) more productive compared to those in nonprimary care roles.

This study gives one example of the many factors to consider when exploring productivity. Other factors include population density, facility capacity, support staffing, procedures performed, research roles, and other nonclinical responsibilities.

Compensation-to-Production Ratio

In the analysis of an operating margin, the compensation paid to providers becomes an important factor. Provider productivity as related to provider compensation more clearly defines the actual cost of the productivity. Total compensation may include salary, bonus, incentives, and honoraria. Physician compensation is significantly more than either PAs or NPs, so direct compensation comparisons are unbalanced and should be considered with productivity measures.

In a study of family medicine physicians, PAs and NPs, the compensation-to-production ratio was measured based on data from the Medical Group Management Association (MGMA) 2014 Physician Compensation & Production Survey Based on 2013 Data (Essary, Green, & Gans, 2016). Mean annual compensation was compared to total patient encounters for 1,734 physicians, 176 NPs, and 95 PAs in MGMA member physician group practices. Providers were all in full-time family medicine practice without obstetrics. Average compensation was equivalent for PAs and NPs ($100,981 and $99,731, respectively) compared to $230,884 for physicians. PAs and physicians reported similar annual patient encounters (3,933 and 3,908, respectively) compared to 2,886 for NPs. The family medicine compensation-to-production ratios based on this data were as follows:

Physicians: 58.70

PAs: 25.84

NPs: 34.56

Keeping in mind that practice setting, geographical location, and other factors influence productivity as well, using compensation-to-production ratio formulas is more informative in comparing productivity among provider professions.

EVALUATION CRITERIA

To provide sustainable health care delivery, the health care system must remain financially viable. As today's market forces require proactive and frequent adjustments to regulatory change while advancing relevant and progressive health care services, staying vigilant to economic factors is critical for the APP leader. However, revenue and cost measures cannot be considered in a vacuum. The performance outcomes of an organization must include measures of financial fortitude in combination with the efficiency of care and, most importantly, the outcome measures of improved health of those served and their satisfaction with services provided. The value of cost-effective care cannot be limited to only the gain or loss of income.

A cluster of outcome measures is necessary to fully evaluate the performance of a health care system. In Case Study 1, Chelsea is challenged by unsatisfactory results of a single factor related to costs associated with higher utilization of ancillary services. However, this factor in isolation from the other measures, particularly when comparing performance outcomes with other comparable clinics, does not fairly address the surrounding conditions. Analyzing financial outcomes should be in conjunction with all performance criteria. One example of a comprehensive evaluation system is the Baldrige Evaluation Criteria (Baldrige Performance Excellence Program, 2017). This system provides an extensive system of evaluation structured for health care organizations across three domains: leadership, performance, and results.

» **Leadership domain:** This domain includes measures of senior leadership effectiveness, governance and societal responsibilities, strategic development and implementation, and patient engagement.

» **Performance domain:** Factors measure knowledge management and performance improvement, workforce engagement and environment, and work processes.

» **Results domain:** The results measured include outcomes of health care, customer satisfaction, finances, workforce satisfaction and process, and leadership effectiveness.

A well-developed evaluation of performance measures that encompasses the mission and values of the health care system will identify the success of the organization.

CASE STUDY 1 (CONTINUED)

After meeting with the APP peers across the retail-based clinics, Chelsea realized that none of the options the CFO offered would be effective. The feedback from the APPs also helped her recognize that from the APPs' point of view, she needed to bring an entirely different approach to consider the concerns raised about the utilization of lab and x-ray. Her proposal to the CFO 2 weeks later went as follows:

After discussions with the APP staff, I have four recommendations to propose in response to the concerns raised by the company over the higher rate of utilization of the ancillary lab and x-ray services compared to the physician-based clinics:

1. *Analyze APP wRVU data: We would like to revisit the data on the APP productivity using wRVUs instead of patient volume to gain a more accurate measure of the work performed.*

2. *Quality Payment Program Participation: We have selected several activities that fit the merit-based incentive payments available for practice sites in the areas of quality care measures and quality improvement measures. This will generate incentive payments that should offset the costs of any overage in the use of the ancillary services for this next year.*

3. *Initiate new marketing strategy: We recommend a new marketing strategy that offers our acute primary care services to the local Medicare population who do not yet have a medical home. Our message will focus on meeting their immediate health care needs while helping them establish routine care with a local clinical practice. By an addition of $5,000 to our budget, this marketing campaign will appeal to this audience, serve as a gateway for greater access to care, and increase our patient volume.*

4. *Revisit performance measures: We recommend a different approach to explore the productivity measures of our clinics and offer to help redesign this strategy to address the following:*

   a. *Include compensation-to-production ratios if comparisons are made to physician-based practices.*

b. *Add a measure of actual patient outcomes of improved health in addition to patient satisfaction.*

c. *Avoid using one factor as an independent indicator of clinical success.*

d. *When comparing productivity measures between clinics and providers, analyze and compare all factors.*

We believe these strategies will help us build on the strengths of our clinics and the care we provide to our communities. We look forward to exploring these recommendations with you.

In Case Study 1, Chelsea chose to avoid voicing the criticisms raised by her APP team. She expresses herself with an understanding of health care economics (application of wRVU, implementation of QPP, and addressing productivity outcomes). Her proposal is forward-thinking, addressing core values of her team (high-quality care, improved patient health outcomes, increased access to care) with practical applications.

Chelsea added a marketing initiative that targets a specific population with a clear message at a reasonable cost to support a professional and high-quality message consistent with the reputation of the clinical services and goals. In any health care system that serves consumers, a carefully planned marketing strategy is necessary.

MARKETING STRATEGIES

In today's market-driven culture, the local health care organization must attend to announcing services offered to reach the population it intends to serve. To be sustainable, the organization is dependent on generating income; strategies must send the right message to the right people.

Marketing programs carry significant risk. A message that is misinterpreted as self-serving or greedy, too flashy, too dull, unclear, or confusing will do more harm than good. Therefore, it is advisable to consider a reasonable investment in the marketing plan, including the services of a marketing consultant skilled at conveying the mission of the organization to the target audience. An objective understanding of consumer opinion and external market forces across the community prior to launching a program is one benefit of securing a consultant to assist with the strategy. A health care organization's public messaging should be distinguishable from other sales strategies that flood the market by following these recommendations:

» Maintain a high level of professionalism

» Avoid jingles, discounts, or competitive language

» Address core values of the health care organization

» Focus the message on meeting health care needs, serving those in need of care

APPs AND FINANCIAL MANAGEMENT

The APP leader need not hold sole responsibility for the financial management of the organization's health care delivery but must be cognizant that high-quality health care cannot be provided without fiscally responsible direction. The APP leader is able to make a significant contribution of perspective and practical application to make necessary financial decisions.

SUMMARY POINTS

1. The APP functions in a health care system dependent on responsible financial management. The APP is able to practice more knowledgably with an understanding of the services of the health care system that maintains high-quality health care delivery, each with its own costs. Effective financial management requires budgeting strategies tailored to meet the needs of different areas across the organization. Recognizing decentralized budgeting processes brings opportunities to help explore financial implications that affect the local health care team. Budgeting processes are influenced by the APP leader to improve cost-effective care using zero-based, incremental, performance-based, or responsibility-centered budgeting models. Maximizing the operating margin depends on familiarity with various revenue streams such as pay-for-service, DRG and global payments, RVUs and participation in quality payment programs.

2. Productivity outcomes are vital to determining sustainable, cost-effective health care delivery. APP leaders should help guide the selection of performance measures that represent the unique environment of the local health care organization. The number of patient encounters, wRVUs, patient outcomes, or other factors measure productivity. Comparisons of work and cost such as compensation-to-production ratios are likely more meaningful and should be combined with a balance of other outcome measures (e.g., leadership effectiveness, workforce engagement, health care outcomes, and patient satisfaction) in making financially sound decisions.

3. It may seem convenient to leave financial concerns to accountants and business managers; however, they need the perspective of the health care provider. APP leaders must help guide decisions on financial management of the health care system by contributing their expertise to enhance the health care team and maintain the needed focus on high-quality patient care. Two examples where APP leader engagement offers critical input are in the evaluation of performance measures and the development of marketing strategies.

REFERENCES

Baldrige Performance Excellence Program. (2017). *2017–2018 Baldrige excellence framework (health care): A systems approach to improving your organization's performance.* Gaithersburg, MD: National Institute of Standards and Technology.

Essary, A. C., Green, E. P., & Gans, D. N. (2016). Compensation and production in family medicine by practice ownership. *Health Services Research and Managerial Epidemiology.* doi:10.1177/2333392815624111

Mathauer, I., & Wittenbecher, F. (2013). Hospital payment systems based on diagnosis-related groups: Experiences in low- and middle-income countries. *Bulletin of the World Health Organization, 91*, 746–756A.

Medical Group Management Association. (2014). *Physician compensation & production survey, 2014 Report based on 2013 data.* Englewood, CO: Medical Group Management Association.

Moran, E. A., Basa, E., Gao, J., Woodmansee, D., Almenoff, P. L., & Hooker, R. S. (2016). PA and NP productivity in the Veterans Health Administration. *American Academy of Physician Assistants, 29*(7). doi:10.1097/01 .JAA.0000484311.96684.0c

Pickard, T. (2014). Calculating your worth: Understanding productive and value. *Journal of the Advanced Practitioner in Oncology, 5*(2), 128–133.

8

CHANGE STRATEGIES IN HEALTH CARE

CRITICAL THINKING QUESTIONS

» **What can a leader do to achieve change in complex health care systems?**

» **How should the advanced practice provider (APP) respond to resistance to change?**

» **What methods are more effective for the APP to lead implementation of change in health care delivery?**

The adage, "Change never starts because change never stops," has never been truer. Health care evolution and particularly the recent years of health policy reform have brought combinations of hope and frustration because of the never-ending changes constantly at hand. Efforts at regulation and deregulation, social and political sway, new pathogens, greater technology, medical research discoveries, and opportunities to solve global health care issues require nimbleness and adaptability. There is no respite from change in health care delivery.

Acknowledging that change is inevitable brings to focus the need for change to be efficient and for the better. The APP cannot be static in this world of change and must be willing to help guide the change. APP leaders are able to influence change to reach desired goals.

In health care teams, the forms of change fall into one of the following six areas (Yukl, 2013):

Roles: Job redesigns, schedule adjustments, modifying workflow processes, and changing protocols all lead to changes in roles of team responsibilities.

Attitudes: Use of team-building activities or cultural sensitivity training are examples of efforts to change attitudes. These often stem from resistance to change; such efforts help the team become positive forces of change. A change in role typically brings a change in attitude and together may be the path to a more constructive, progressive work environment.

Technology: Implementing new software management systems, and then further adapting these systems as health care organizations grow and expand, require technology change. Electronic medical records is an example experienced by virtually all APPs in clinical practice. Technology change more widely includes an array of information resources, electronic communication vehicles, medical devices, and health care outcome measures that are obligatory to all organizations delivering health care. The goal of technology change is higher efficiency and greater accuracy. This may depend on successful changes in roles and attitudes accompanying the change in technology.

Strategy: Strategic planning is integral to any organization's growth and development, and becomes the plan for change. Identifying new avenues for meeting health care needs, adapting to patient markets, advancing the quality of health care, and adjusting to regulation revisions are common areas that require strategy change (see further discussion later in this chapter).

Economics: Balancing the organization's costs with revenue, local and national economic issues, and continuing to stay financially solvent if not earn a profit brings requirements for internal change (see Chapter 7).

People: Efforts to maximize human potential require a focus on what personnel changes are necessary within the health care team. While this category of change has to address reductions-in-force (when economic change is required), it also applies positively to opportunities to expand services.

These categories of change offer examples that show how change in one area is often a result of, or leads to, change in another area. The sustainability of today's health care systems, from small rural clinics to tertiary care centers, is dependent on the ability to adapt to this environment of predictable and unpredictable change. Anticipating change at every turn in a health care system, the APP must be vigilant to determine when and if change is needed.

CASE STUDY 1

Bella is a nurse practitioner working with a nonprofit clinic for a medical mission agency in an inner-city environment. The mission agency has asked her team to revisit their long-standing mission statement: "Excellence in care with a spirit of compassion." The agency leaders suggested that the statement was in need of a fresh look.

Excited to be tasked with bringing the team together to explore the mission statement, Bella gathered the eight staff and key volunteers to develop a recommendation for the next era of the clinic's outreach. She scheduled an afternoon meeting to include a team-building activity, followed by a brainstorming session to find key words and phrases that represent the team's vision for the future. From that session, she planned to facilitate a concluding discussion to bring those terms together into a pithy, contemporary mission statement proposal.

After a fun outdoors activity, her team assembled and began to explore terms that emulated their clinic's services and goals, writing ideas on white boards for all to see. Not long into the activity, Bella found the team stalled over searching for words that were synonyms for "excellence," "care," and "compassion." One of the team then said, "I'm not sure what's wrong with our current mission statement."

After further discussion, the team expressed a clear, renewed commitment to the existing mission statement. In unanimous agreement, Bella planned to report to the mission agency leadership that the team was revitalized by the mission statement review and recommended no changes.

THREE STAGES OF CHANGE

Change process theories abound, but they typically center on three steps originally presented by Kurt Lewin in the 1950s. Called the "force field model," its premise shares the theme of Newton's third law of motion: for every action there is an equal and opposite reaction. In the middle, some type of equilibrium is sustained. Lewin called this the state of "quasi-stationary equilibrium."

In any situation of change, there are those seeking change and those wanting to keep things as they are. The equilibrium reached between these two forces balances the status quo. This is the force field, and change can occur only by two means: increasing conditions that favor the change or reducing the resistance to change.

In this model, Lewin presents a three-stage theory of change (Lewin, 1951): Unfreeze, change, and refreeze (see Figure 8.1). In organizational management, some find this theory overly simplistic in light of the complexities of today's world (to be addressed later in this chapter), but these three stages serve as a foundation for understanding change. As described subsequently, each stage requires planning prior to implementation.

1. **Unfreeze**

    This stage requires a thoughtful determination that old ways are inadequate. A crisis abruptly brings this stage of unfreeze; it is then

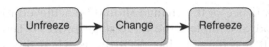

FIGURE 8.1 Lewin's three-stage theory of change.
Source: Adapted from Lewin (1951).

immediately clear that a current process is failing. More often in health care teams, there is a discovery of opportunities or challenges that provoke new directions. Typically, this first surfaces within an individual or a few team members. It is important the team all understand and appreciate the depth of the opportunity or challenge at this stage.

If change occurs without this opportunity to unfreeze, the team will bring resistance or become apathetic and not be devoted to making the change work. Many consider this stage most important for the reasons illustrated in Case Study 1. Bella's team, energized by the appeal of designing a new mission statement, soon recognized in initial discussions (the unfreeze stage) that the need for change was unclear and perhaps not necessary.

2. **Change**

   In Lewin's theory, this stage is not a one-time event but a process. It is the hardest stage as while the team may all favor the change, the actual experience of change brings uncertainty and doubt. To help alleviate those concerns, there must be a clear process of transition to implement change. When possible, the team should study more than one proposal for change and solve anticipated obstacles. This requires time, which is not always available. The team should agree on the most promising course to follow.

   If attention to this stage is avoided or change is implemented hastily, the transition is weakened and more likely to fail.

3. **Refreeze**

   This stage occurs upon full implementation of the change and establishes the "new normal." Though the adjustments are still fragile, the team accepts the change and in this stage becomes comfortable in the new system. This takes time, sometimes a significant length of time, which is why Lewin's model receives criticism by those in health care systems. In today's complex environment, the next change may need implementation before this refreezing is complete. Lewin has argued that permanence of the change should be achieved for at least some time period to complete the three-stage process (Lewin, 1947). The evidence that refreezing has occurred is when the team's dynamic returns to an effective, functional level.

Change without refreezing brings a loss of consensus favoring the change, resulting in diminished enthusiasm. If not addressed, the risk of change reversal is high, returning to old ways.

Actions to Achieve Change

Lewin recommends two actions to achieve change in this model. First, the benefits of the change should be clear if not tangible, such as setting rewards for accomplishing the transition. The change may bring a natural benefit, but anticipating the transition is often difficult. Sweetening the desired outcome with incentives helps maintain the motivation of the team as change agents. Secondly, the concerns of the resistant should be reduced by minimizing fears, addressing concerns of failure or other economic worries. If the resistance is strong, exploring ways to remove the opposition may be required.

Either action may be useful, and the initial force field analysis predicts what is needed based on the strength of the team favoring the change against the forces of resistance. If opposition is strong, fully employ both actions.

CASE STUDY 1 (CONTINUED)

Bella returned to the mission agency leadership to report that the existing mission statement, "Excellence in care with a spirit of compassion," was studied and no recommendations for change were made. She announced that her team renewed their commitment to the current mission statement as holding relevance and guidance in setting their course for the future.

The leadership respected the team's conclusion and gave Bella further direction. Agreeing to support the existing mission statement, they asked Bella to develop a plan to evaluate outcomes to demonstrate the mission statement was being achieved.

With this refined directive, Bella developed a more extensive plan of study. She created a proposal to include a series of meetings with her team over the next few months, first to explore what outcomes were measurable to meet the expectations of "excellent care" and "compassion." She then planned to distribute assignments among her team to develop tools and processes capturing data that would reflect these measures. In her timeline, the implementation of the measures would occur in 4 months and require a data collection period of at least 6 months. After a period of analysis, she would then present the leadership with outcomes to determine if the clinic's mission statement was being achieved.

Bella planned to return her proposal to the leadership with two requests if the proposal was accepted. One, she would ask the agency to support a 1-day retreat for her team at the midway point of her proposal just prior to the data collection period. The retreat, hosted at the lakeside camp of the mission agency, would be a reward for the team's efforts, including time for team development as well as personal reflection. Secondly, the agency would provide assurance that if the outcomes did not meet their benchmarks of success, there would be no threat of loss of funding or personnel.

Bella's strategy in meeting the agency's request for measuring mission statement–directed outcomes follows the Lewin model for establishing change. The initial meetings to explore what outcomes are measurable and developing appropriate tools represent a period of unfreezing. She has planned a 6-month period of data collection, the actual change itself. She has minimized the threat of this change by asking for a promise that upon learning the results, no negative actions would result during the period of refreezing (accepting the evaluation of the team in meeting the mission as the new norm). She has also negotiated for an incentive by the 1-day retreat for the team to enjoy midway through the transition process.

RESISTANCE TO CHANGE

According to Lewin's force field model, there will always be resistance to change; it is expected. Healthy and respectable resistance is not due to ignorance or inflexibility, and the APP leader should welcome the insights of the resistors. Addressing the concerns raised and identifying obstacles allow time for planned responses to challenges that would otherwise surface during the second stage (change). This valuable interaction may convert opponents to change, leading to heightened motivation and the increased energy needed for success.

Responsible reasons to resist change deserve attention and should be raised if evident. See Table 8.1 for examples in challenging change. Each example requires a response of clarification. If the leader cannot reasonably defend the change against the claim, reconsider the need for change.

TABLE 8.1 Reasons to Resist Change

Conflicts with ideals/principles

High-cost/low-benefit ratio

Not needed

Not practical

Result will cause significant loss (income, personnel, autonomy, etc.)

Success is doubtful

For example, a proposed change would streamline the current process of patient lab results callbacks, saving the APPs valuable time by replacing patient phone calls with electronic notification. The proposal would eliminate approximately 85% of the phone calls now required, avoiding missed calls, and promising a more timely delivery of normal lab results. Reasonable concerns include whether the APPs are expected to schedule additional patients to replace the time saved in the phone calls or if the proposal intends to alleviate the burden of the callbacks (consideration of how the change would personally affect each APP). Will patients view this change as disrupting a commitment to personalized clinician–patient communication (inconsistent with values)? Such questions serve only to refine the change process, guiding the team to success.

Sources of Power in Change Strategies

APP leaders utilize various sources of power when helping the team deliberate on change. Legitimate, referent, expert, and coercion powers all are at the leader's disposal (see Chapter 2).

Legitimate power: Communicating the rationale for the change, reasoning with the team regarding the benefits and risks of change. "Here's why it makes sense."

Referent power: Calling the team toward the shared value system that supports the change. "We believe this is the right thing to do."

Expert power: Identifying how the team is prepared with the appropriate experience and foundation to implement the change with the right people in position. "We are uniquely qualified to lead this change."

Coercion power: If resistance persists after exhausting the aforementioned power sources and this new direction is clearly right, the leader may have to call the team to action. "We've just got to do this."

CHANGE FATIGUE

In the complexities of today's health care systems, change occurs with a high rate of frequency. Many changes in direct patient care lead to enhanced diagnostic or treatment modalities, more satisfying clinician and patient experiences, and improved patient outcomes. In the midst of these positive changes are ongoing Medicare and other regulatory changes, institution of quality control measures, and new provisions for patient safety or liability protection. Health care systems that are not involved in an abundance of change are likely falling behind.

In this environment, some find that repeated change builds resilience, particularly if the changes are regularly successful processes. The team is more willing to take risks when there is a history of beneficial change. The term "change fatigue" indicates a loss of this resiliency. When the team is fatigued with change, they are more vulnerable to languish in the inherent and difficult challenges of change. The persistent stress of uncertainty wears out the team with less enthusiasm, a loss of motivation, and increased sick days (Hansson, Vingård, Arnetz, & Anderzén, 2008).

Change fatigue among health care workers is different from resistance to change (McMillan & Perron, 2013). The latter is an intentional decision to confront change, compared to change fatigue as a lived experience in response to repeated change. Resistance to change is not associated with absenteeism or increased sick days. While there is little benefit to change fatigue, change resistance in small doses stimulates critical thinking and offers anticipation of consequences. Resistance to change is typically active and vocal; change fatigue is passive and may go unnoticed.

Using a more elaborate process to evaluate a change strategy will identify obstacles to change, including change fatigue. The action research model presented herein is one example of a planned change process.

PLANNED CHANGE IN COMPLEX HEALTH CARE ENVIRONMENTS

In responding to the complex and often turbulent health care environment, a more extensive process to develop planned change is required. Within the scope of a lean, highly functioning health care team, the three-stage theory of change offers a framework to manage common issues. In a health care system with multiple interacting units that are dynamic within a commonly labyrinthine structure, change faces unique challenges that are difficult to predict. A review of historical and contextual factors is required. A cross-sectional survey at one point in time is likely insufficient to determine the best direction for change; more intensive study to explore relationships and overlapping or concurrent processes is necessary. Models of change may need testing via computer simulation or consultation with comparable organizations who have conducted similar transitions are in order. The action research model is a classic, cyclical process that engages a focused study (research) of the organization and environmental factors to guide the change (action).

CASE STUDY 2

Ben is a physician assistant (PA), one of 20 APPs employed by a multispecialty clinic in a suburban community of 300,000 people. He works with five general internists, and the practice houses eight related internal medicine subspecialties with 25 physicians. Raised in this community, Ben has settled here with his wife and three children.

The primary practice has recently enjoyed significant growth, adding three physicians last year and a plan to add two more on residency completion this year. The administration has announced a goal of hiring at least one APP for every physician, and each of three cardiologists already has two APPs providing direct patient care on their specialty service.

The practice opened two urgent care clinics in the past 18 months, designed to meet immediate primary care needs of adult patients with the goal of funneling these individuals to a patient-centered medical home in the primary practice. The urgent care clinics' patient volume is high, staffed with APPs from the primary practice on a rotating schedule. Physicians staff the urgent care clinics one or two afternoons a week. Earlier this year the clinic opened an aesthetics clinic, now boasting a remarkable performance, staffed with three full-time APPs and a dermatologist.

At the annual end-of-year employee banquet, the clinic celebrated these successes with generous bonuses given to all clinical staff including the APPs. The medical director presented an overview of the past year's success and outlined the 5-year plan for future growth. For the first time the employees heard plans to add three new subspecialties to the practice with construction of an additional floor to their present building. In addition, the director announced an upcoming groundbreaking ceremony for a new freestanding surgical center to be eventually staffed with five surgeons. Lastly, the third and fourth, new urgent care clinics are scheduled to open over the next 2 years.

At the banquet, Ben and his wife were amazed with this whirlwind of growth and expansion. They sensed an excitement around the room in light of the progressive advancement of their clinic to expand services and further meet the health care needs of their community.

As Ben was leaving the banquet, he passed a cluster of five of his APP peers near the exit. He quickly found that they did not share his enthusiasm for the plans of growth.

"What'd you think of all that mess?" one of the APPs said to him.

"Certainly, there's a lot going on right now," Ben cautiously responded.

"We were just talking about it. We don't think we want to be part of this cash cow anymore. They've lost their focus; all they want to do is grow, grow, grow." The others in the circle nodded, adding their own grumblings.

Another one said, "I'm going to have to look at what else is out there. This isn't what I signed up for. They can find another lackey for this job; it isn't going to be me."

Ben leaves, shocked by what he has heard. He admires his APP peers and didn't realize before now that others were this discouraged with their employment. He's sure the management team is unaware.

What role should Ben play in trying to address the concerns of his peers?

SYSTEMS PERSPECTIVE

In Case Study 2, Ben is confronted with a budding revolt among his peers against planned change in the form of the growth and expansion of the multispecialty clinic he works for.

The scope of this change has ramifications far beyond his APP peers or a single health care team. The health care organization is an open system in constant interaction with many facets across the community and state. The role of the individual APP seems only a small component of a much larger machine. However, all functions of the organization are interrelated, so that consequences of growth are difficult to limit to a confined area. A beneficial change or an unfavorable inefficiency in one area of the organization will eventually affect others. Ben's APP peers are challenged by this planned expansion, but likely do not grasp the scope of the organization's goals. Neither do they feel the organization is in line with their own motivations.

The APP leader must appreciate the purpose and value of the administrative leadership. Any sizable organization must be led by an administrative team with the following goals:

» **Increase organizational capacity:** measured by the agility, health, and effectiveness of the organization.

» **Improve individuals and relationships:** supporting the development of skills and positive attitudes that contribute to productive interactions and successful problem solving.

» **Manage change:** acknowledging that change is continual, planned as much as possible, and contributes to long-range goals.

» **Shape organizational culture:** upholding the values and beliefs adopted by the organization as evidenced by both behaviors and outcomes.

The final item in the list about organizational culture is key to the success of the administrative leadership. To support successful adaptations and improvements, the organizational culture must be clear and managed well, linked to an effective business strategy. Organizational culture predicts success or failure in today's unsettled health care environment.

Organizational Culture

The elements of organizational culture have been identified as artifacts, norms, values, and basic assumptions (Schein, 2010):

» **Artifacts:** highly visible symbols indicative of deeper cultural values, including day-to-day behaviors, dress, and language.

» **Norms:** unspoken rules that represent how the team members interact with each other, such as the use of first names or last names when addressing co-workers or always addressing a physician as "doctor" rather than by the first name.

» **Values:** the values in use, not necessarily posted, that place importance on what the organization believes deserves attention. For example, when needing to stay late to see patients at the clinic, these values become clear in determining if staff needs hold priority over patient needs or the reverse.

» **Basic assumptions:** intrinsic beliefs that represent how team members think. These are nonnegotiable principles that apply to all relationships in the work environment. Basic assumptions are the foundation for the values, norms, and artifacts of the organizational culture. The inherent dignity of all people would be an esteemed basic assumption.

As shown in Figure 8.2A, the elements of organizational culture are interrelated, building up from the core of basic assumptions. Artifacts, while clearly visible, are subtle indications of norms that reflect the operational values that stem from the basic assumptions.

To illustrate the interactive function of the organizational culture elements, Figure 8.2B provides a bipolar example of each element level. One basic assumption in an organization is the source of knowledge: either

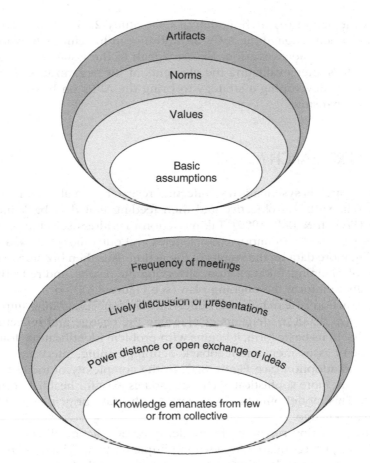

FIGURE 8.2A AND 8.2B Elements of organizational culture, Model-A, Applied-B.

it comes from the collective or from a few in leadership. At the level of values, the collective embraces the exchange of ideas, while knowledge from a few more likely supports power distance leadership (leaders who make decisions at a distance from the rest of the team). The norms are represented by lively discussions during staff meetings in the collective, while meetings are likely directive presentations if knowledge is from a few. Artifacts would reflect these norms, values, and the basic assumptions by the frequency of meetings (more often if knowledge is from the collective, fewer if knowledge is from a few).

With this understanding of the administrative goals of a health care organization and the intricacies of organizational culture, the complexities of planned change require a more elaborate developmental strategy, such as the action research model. In Case Study 2, Ben is in a singular position to help engage the APPs around him in his clinic's transition to further growth and expansion. He can speak to the issues raised by the APP resistors after evaluating the elements of the organizational culture of the clinic, developing a strategy to bring the APPs on board with the planned expansion.

ACTION RESEARCH MODEL

Action research is systematically collecting research data about an ongoing system relative to an objective and then feeding that data back into the system (French & Bell, 1999). Taking action that alters selected variables in the system seeks to improve efficiencies and outcomes as measured by collecting more data on the results of the action. This then becomes a cyclic process of planning, taking action, observing the results, and reflecting on the results to inform the ongoing plan (see Figure 8.3).

The action research model builds on this concept, adding important steps to give detail to elements of planning the change and reflecting on the results. In its basic form, it begins with problem identification, followed by a cycle of assessment and feedback, action planning, intervention, evaluation, and adoption (see Figure 8.4). In the complexity of today's health care systems, more sophisticated change models exist for health care administrators. This model offers a framework to illustrate principles addressed in strategic change.

True to action research, the model integrates action directed by the research, requiring collaboration with multiple partners. The ongoing need for data collection and analysis requires a team to both diagnose and solve

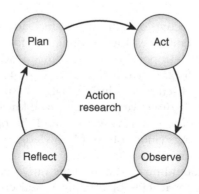

FIGURE 8.3 Action research.

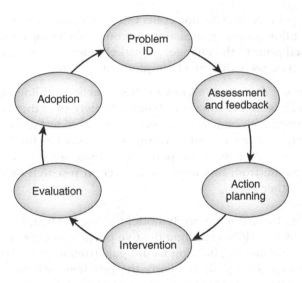

FIGURE 8.4 Action research model.

problems. When it functions cyclically, the organization's ability to solve future problems can be maximized.

» **Problem identification:** This is the most critical but most neglected stage. It requires an assessment of the team's readiness for change. In Case Study 3, Ben has recognized that the APPs were not ready for more change, and change fatigue was apparent. After the problem is clarified with the rationale for the change, ownership of the need for change may develop. This brings a commitment on the part of the team to support the change. Jumping past this stage too quickly leads to conflict and obstructions later if the team is not prepared for the change intervention.

» **Assessment and feedback:** Various types of measures are deployed here, such as surveys, questionnaires, focus group interviews, and other observations. Reviewing documents related to performance and outcomes informs the team in preparation for developing the action plan.

» **Action planning:** The action plan is created based on the goals for the change. At this stage, implications are determined, including time requirements, financial costs, personnel support, and physical/environmental needs. Exploring the consequences of the change, including potential gains and losses, offers guidance to developing action plan details.

» **Intervention:** At this stage, the actual change is implemented. Its success is dependent on the work completed with each previous step of the model.

» **Evaluation:** New data are collected to measure the success of the intervention and to remeasure outcomes for comparison with data analyzed prior to the change. All stakeholders participate in the evaluation process with a newly implemented change.

» **Adoption:** This stage allows further practice, adding necessary enhancements to fine-tune the change. Anxiety over the change should be reduced with benefits duly noted, reported as "success stories," to encourage the team. Positive results lead toward institutionalization of the change. Over time, the period of adoption expires and the team can separate from this focus of the action research model and turn toward other needs.

Applying the action research model to Case Study 2, Ben should consider gathering the APPs, including the five peers who expressed resistance to the clinic's expansion. The team would gain from together processing the proposed change, beginning to clarify the problem, evaluating the degree of change fatigue, and seeking greater ownership of the change, all features of the first stage of the model.

For Ben's leadership to be effective, he needs to be thoughtful in his approach to his team. The model of strategic thinking may be helpful to guide his next steps.

STRATEGIC LEADERSHIP

Two strategies to explore change are strategic planning and strategic thinking (see Table 8.2). *Strategic planning* is the participatory process the team undergoes to examine the future and determine, for the team or institutionally,

TABLE 8.2 Strategic Planning Versus Strategic Thinking

Strategic Planning	Strategic Thinking
Regimented	Creative
Smooth	Disruptive
Reality-focused	Future-focused
Tested	Experimental
Bureaucratic	Systems perspective
Financially driven	Intent-driven
Analytic	Hypothetical

in what direction to head. It is important to plan change whenever possible to prevent the team from becoming reactionary to environmental influences.

With strategic planning, the team creates its own future. The goals of strategic planning should be set for a 3- to 5-year period, including measurable, achievable results within 1 to 2 years. Framed as an event, strategic planning is a critical component in the process of planned change.

Strategic thinking is required of the leader to determine *how* to achieve strategic planning. Strategic thinking is creative; the leader explores many directions, allowing ideas to be disruptive if not outlandish at this stage of exploration. While putting the plan in place must be based on reality, strategic thinking is future-oriented, exploring possible utopian advantages as well as tough deterrents.

While strategic planning must be orderly, going through channels of approval, strategic thinking can manipulate the system without boundaries. The leader can consider the impact of change from any direction and may wish to develop mental scenarios of alternative futures to test out the resiliency of the change. Strategic planning must consider financial implications, but strategic thinking is not beholden to such constraints.

Strategic thinking can start with the questions, How can we be better? How can we reach farther? The strategic leader does well to explore these questions. Strategic thinking is then hypothetical and planning must be more analytical.

Returning to Case Study 2, Ben may find through strategic thinking that he can clarify the clinic's future-focused, intent-driven advancements from a systems perspective. Bringing the team of APPs together to explore these directions in the context of their own needs may better define the reasons for resistance. If resistance persists, bringing thoughtful concerns forward to the administration is only helpful to achieve the clinic's overall growth and expansion.

IMPLEMENTING CHANGE

At the point of making the change, researchers debate whether it is best to implement the transition gradually or rapidly. Fast change prevents organized resistance, though evidence suggests that gradual change is more successful. Amis, Slack, and Hinings (2004) reported on a study of 36 national sports organizations in Canada between 1984 and 1996. They found that radical changes were more successful when messages about the importance of the change were highly visible, followed by a persistent, dedicated, and serious process of change. Their study noted that the path of gradual change was inconsistent and nonlinear. Anticipated delays offered opportunities to make adjustments. At times, the process was even temporarily reversed to make concessions, win collaborations, and deploy beneficial modifications.

While the APP leader needs to consider the unique environment around him or her in planning change (see Exercise 8.1), the strategy surrounding a gradual implementation is advised.

EXERCISE 8.1 QUESTIONS FOR THE STRATEGIC LEADER

In this application of strategic thinking, the APP leader sets time aside to explore the following series of questions. The answers offer a framework for developing a plan for change using Lewin's three-stage theory of change or the action research model.

1. *How did we get where we are today?*

2. *What's accounted for our success (or lack thereof)?*

3. *Where do we want to go?*

4. *Are our strengths supportive of the mission?*

5. *How do we get to where we want to go?*

6. *What are the critical risks?*

7. *What are the key results?*

SUMMARY POINTS

1. With the pressure of market forces and regulatory demands bearing down on every health care system, change is an expectation, at times rapid, unexpected, and consistently frequent. At a minimum, the steps of unfreeze, change, and refreeze (Lewin's three-stage theory of change) are necessary to implement effective change. The APP must be nimble and readily adjust to what feels like instability in the health care system. By staying abreast of change, if not helping to lead it, the APP leader helps the organization advance, likely finding improved outcomes for patient care. The APP can help achieve the planned changes by two actions: clarifying for the team the benefits of change and responding to the concerns of those resisting the change, the latter by addressing concerns of failure.

2. Change always faces some degree of resistance; engaging the contrary parties refines the transition process. Acknowledging resistance as healthy allows the APP to consider the concerns raised, identify the obstacles, and develop solutions ahead of time that otherwise may

later be caustic to achieving the goals of the change. Resisting change may be in order to give time to address opportunities to improve the implementation process. If the team is not ready for change, caution is exercised in moving forward. APPs may find legitimate, referent, and expert powers of use in leading change. If the resistance to change is strong or change fatigue is an issue, a more elaborate process of change strategy is necessary.

3. The action research model provides a framework for change strategy in a complex environment such as today's health care systems. Starting with a focus on problem identification, the model continues in a cycle of assessment and feedback, action planning, intervention, evaluation, and adoption. Attention to each step of the cycle keeps the APP in a position to anticipate challenges and solve obstacles. When the APP leader has the opportunity to set the course for advancement, a focused process of strategic thinking will provide the guidance needed to bring the team together for successful transitions.

REFERENCES

Amis, J., Slack, T., & Hinings, C. R. (2004). The pace, sequence and linearity of radical change. *The Academy of Management Journal, 47*(1) 15–39.

French, W. L., & Bell, C. H. (1999). *Organizational development: Behavioral science interventions for organization improvement* (6th ed.). Upper Saddle River, NJ: Pearson.

Hansson, A., Vingård, E., Arnetz, B. B., & Anderzén, I. (2008). Organizational change, health, and sick leave among health care employees: A longitudinal study measuring stress markers, individual, and work site factors. *Work & Stress, 22*(1), 69–80.

Lewin, K. (1947). Frontiers in group dynamics: Concept, method and reality in social science; social equilibria and social change. *Human Relations, 1*, 5–40.

Lewin, K. (1951). *Field theory in social science.* New York, NY: Harper & Row.

McMillan, K., & Perron, A. (2013). Nurses amidst change: The concept of change fatigue offers an alternative perspective on organizational change. *Policy, Politics & Nursing Practice, 14*(1), 26–32.

Schein, E. (2010). *Organizational culture and leadership* (4th ed.). San Francisco, CA: Jossey-Bass.

Yukl, G. (2013). *Leadership in organizations* (8th ed., pp. 77–81). Upper Saddle River, NJ: Pearson.

PART 3
The Human Aspects of Clinical Leadership

ETHICS AND THE CULTURALLY INFORMED CLINICAL LEADER

CRITICAL THINKING QUESTIONS

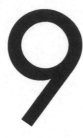

9
ETHICS AND THE CULTURALLY
INFORMED CLINICAL LEADER

CRITICAL THINKING QUESTIONS

» **Which ethical principles in health care also readily apply to leadership?**

» **When the health care team has disagreements over personally held values, how should the leader respond?**

» **What factors contribute to advancing a health care team to greater intercultural sensitivity?**

» **How can unintentional behaviors provoke misperceptions among the team members about a leader's actions?**

Ethics and culture present two diametrically opposed subjects for leaders. The former, *ethics*, establishes a singular, inarguable, critical standard that every leader is expected to endorse and follow: The leader should uphold the standard of ethical behavior above reproach.

The latter, *culture*, is a widely diverse, multifaceted, intricate concept— individually designed to each leader and every team. It appears differently at every application and varies in definition and measure by each person involved: The leader should embrace cultural diversity to support creativity and social justice.

Both subjects, however, bring the identical challenge to advanced practice provider (APP) leaders. The practice of ethics and engaging culture together can be difficult in the health care environment. They overlap significantly for leaders as each society's culture defines ethics, for good or bad. As an example, the discrimination of individuals in receiving health care is unethical and unacceptable. Choosing who should receive care based on any cultural identifier consistently faces objections, as it should. However, medical triage based on the ability to pay directly reflects on societal culture. Challenges facing the U.S. health care system are tied to subpopulations and their ability to pay, apparent in every form of health care reform dating back to the Medicare/Medicaid initiatives of the 1950s.

DEFINING ETHICS

Ethics should be distinguished from values, morals, and virtues. At its core, ethics is the study and practice of what is good and right. APPs understand the application of ethics in direct patient care is in the context of guiding patients toward choices that uphold accepted moral principles. One's values, morals, and virtues frame her or his ethics.

» **Values:** Enduring principles or deeply held personal beliefs that shape a person's attitudes and behaviors. The "right to life" is an example of a value that directly influences the attitude and behavior of an individual.

» **Morals:** Standards of behaviors based on one's values. "The moral of the story. . ." represents lessons learned by lived experience.

» **Virtues:** Inarguable qualities of moral goodness. Examples that particularly apply to medicine include caring, compassion, trustworthiness, integrity, conscientiousness, and discernment.

When needing to determine the "right" course, the leader will turn to values, morals, and virtues. Ethics that develops from these values, morals, and virtues then answers the question, Why did I follow that course?

ETHICAL PRINCIPLES IN ACTION

Ethical dilemmas occur when the right course is not readily apparent, or when a collision of values exists in exploring the potential solutions to the dilemma. As a leader, a process for considering ethical dilemmas is necessary so one does not lead at the whim of emotion or other pressure. One model for a leader to use in considering ethical dilemmas applies the four ethical principles common to medicine: autonomy, beneficence, justice, and nonmaleficence (Kaldjian, Wier, & Duffy, 2005).

» **Autonomy:** Respect must be granted for the autonomy of the individual(s) facing the dilemma, including their individual goals, desires, and wishes. Agreement may not be reached, but the leader cannot force personal values on another member of the team.

» **Beneficence:** This protects what is best for the individual(s) involved in the dilemma, including a broad perspective of benefits gained physically, emotionally, and socially.

» **Justice:** Justice requires the leader to uphold the legal, financial, cultural, and social norms.

» **Nonmaleficence:** The classic medical phrase "Do no harm" is represented by nonmaleficence. Maintaining nonmaleficence is framed by the facts and accuracy of information involved in the situation surrounding the ethical dilemma.

Together, these ethical principles comprise the "four-box method" of a decision-making matrix (Jonsen, Siegler, & Winsalde, 2015) used to guide a leader in exploring an ethical dilemma (see Table 9.1).

TABLE 9.1 "Four-Box Model" as a Decision-Making Matrix

Nonmaleficence	Autonomy
Includes known facts of the situation	Includes the individual's goals, desires, and wishes
Beneficence	**Justice**
Includes consideration of physical, emotional, and social benefits	Includes legal issues, financial implications, and social norms

CASE STUDY 1

José is a nurse practitioner working in a cardiology group practice in a metropolitan area. He sees patients at the primary site 2 days/week and travels to different communities 3 days/week for ongoing continuous care of patients in those neighboring communities each within a 100-mile radius. José maintains the schedule for himself and three other APPs to manage these clinical sites for the practice. A second team of APPs staff patients as hospitalists in two major hospitals in town, managing their schedule separately within that team.

At the monthly meeting José holds with his team, an ethical concern was raised. With all respect for both teams of APPs, his team working in the outpatient clinics has learned that there is a significant salary differential (estimated at 20%) between the hospitalist APPs and themselves. His team does not believe the differential is justified by experience or education, and they question why the hospitalist APPs earn higher salaries.

His team has brought this forward together, recognizing that the cardiology practice has a clear, written policy that wages and salaries are not to be discussed in comparison among employees. They fear retribution by the administration if they raise their concern, so they are seeking José's leadership in helping to resolve what appears to be a serious inequity.

José tells his team he needs to explore this concern for himself and consider what his response as a leader should be. He employs the four ethical principles from the decision-making matrix.

» **Autonomy:** José respects the privacy of salary information; he himself does not have access to this information. However, he also respects his teammates who feel unfairly compensated. Their concerns deserve an explanation.

» **Beneficence:** While the salary is the point of concern, José believes other questions to ask involve his team members' satisfaction with their professional roles and support. He wonders if there are other work issues brooding beneath the salary concerns.

» **Justice:** There are significant financial implications, and José recognizes that the answer cannot be addressed by a sweep of equalizing salaries. In addition, he must honor the strict policy of not discussing employee salaries; José is aware of a previous occurrence of an employee dismissal over a salary disclosure made to coworkers.

» **Nonmaleficence:** The APPs respect each other and he must preserve this ("do no harm"). A better understanding of the facts is needed. Attempting to validate the salary information is in conflict with the standing confidentiality policy. There are other employment features that need to be considered, such as work hours, on-call hours, intensity of responsibilities, and other requirements of each position that are weighed in determining salaries.

CASE STUDY 1 (CONTINUED)

José returned to his team with information related to the employment issues. All APPs are salaried; no one is paid hourly wages. He shared that the hospitalist APPs all work three 12-hour shifts/week and each person is on a scheduled rotation of day and night shifts. Though they work in interprofessional teams, the hospitalist APPs are called first when an inpatient issue needs to be addressed, including any emergency response, so there is a higher level of intensity expected in their practice.

He presented this information to compare with his team's work schedules. They each staff an 8-hour clinic day at the primary clinic and 7-hour clinic days at the satellite clinics. Travel for the three other clinic days/ week are reimbursed at the federal mileage reimbursement rate, though a corporate vehicle is provided, which is intended to serve as a travel stipend.

José reported that both teams of APPs work more hours than the clinic or hospital shifts dictate, but the increased hours were balanced based on patient volumes in either setting.

He asked his team about other work concerns. While the apparent salary discrepancy was a concern, he invited an open discussion of any other issues related to the team's dissatisfaction with work.

Their response was mostly positive. The physician access and support was in place, the environment and staff support at each location was sufficient, and they generally felt the administration was responsive to needs as they came up. They felt that the travel to the clinics was "getting old," and expressed some frustration over the extra time this took away from their home lives, as they would have to leave home early and return later than clinic days at the primary clinic.

José reminded the team that any further salary comparisons would be outside of their employment policy. He promised to explore this additional information provided today and to get back to them.

Application of the Decision-Making Matrix

José's team meeting provided further insight and direction. Comparing the work schedule provided concrete information. Clarifying these facts for all contributes to nonmaleficence, downplaying any presumptions or potentially baseless accusations. Hearing the team's general affirmation regarding the clinic support gave focus to the salary question. The additional comments on travel discontent were useful, addressing issues of beneficence. His reinforcement of the policy prohibiting salary disclosures respects the autonomy of other APP team members and the principle of justice in honoring the clinic policy.

When the four-box grid is complete, the best approach to resolve a dilemma may be obvious. Other times, the ethical principles are clarified but are in conflict with each other. Arguably, priority may be given to nonmaleficence and autonomy in the decision-making matrix to guide the decision. Ethical decisions based on the facts surrounding the situation are less likely to create harm (nonmaleficence) as they avoid more subjective decision making based on opinions or hearsay. Actions taken in ethical dilemmas that protect the autonomy of individuals are often more defendable and hold support of the team. When an individual's autonomy is respected (as long as that autonomy holds integrity), it is more difficult to question a breach of integrity or equity. In the four-box model, this refers to "staying above the line," referring to the two upper boxes of the model (see Table 9.1).

When applying the two lower boxes of the model, the principles of beneficence and justice are more challenging to uphold. There is typically more subjective opinion involved. Deciding what "good" occurs from beneficence is often individualized based on differing perspectives of physical, emotional, and social norms. As well, various issues of justice can be in conflict, such as legal questions, financial issues, and social culture that do not agree with what seems "right." If an ethical quandary can be solved based on principles of nonmaleficence and autonomy, it likely is a stronger, more secure decision.

José considered the issues framed by the decision-making matrix and approached his administrative leader with a proposal for resolving his team's concern.

CASE STUDY 1 (CONTINUED)

In meeting with the clinic administrator, José provided the information regarding his team's work schedules, patient volume, and travel schedules. He spoke to the team's appreciation for the physician and staff support and the general responsiveness of the administration. He then raised the team's concern (a concern José also held) regarding the disadvantage of the travel time. The travel reimbursement did not sufficiently compensate for the extra time added to the usual work day. Appreciating that there needed to be give and take with the APPs' charting and administrative duties, the fixed travel time roundtrip 3 days/week seemed like a disadvantage to the position.

José offered a couple suggestions to resolve this, such as increasing the compensation so that the travel time was reimbursed at a rate comparable to the salary. He added that with a higher compensation model, the APP would be expected to engage in professional development during 50% of the travel time (e.g., one way during each trip), listening to podcasts or other recordings (at the discretion of the APP) related to professional and medical education. This would allow the travel time to be an investment in the professional development of the APP to the benefit of the practice, and would compensate the APP at a level in respect to the professional role rather than a designated mileage reimbursement.

The alternative suggestion is exploration of hiring an additional APP, perhaps part-time, to cover some of the clinic hours requiring travel so that each APP would work the majority of time at the primary clinic and no

more than 2 days/week traveling to the other communities. José presented a
sample schedule showing how an added APP redistributed the APPs across
the clinics to reduce the individual travel. If the new APP was recruited from
one of the communities, this would reduce travel costs.

José's approach was to entirely avoid the concerns of compensation inequity. He approached the administration with a proposal to address a perceived disadvantage to APPs traveling to clinics, offered two optional solutions, and included a measure of cost savings. This maintained the principle of autonomy for all involved, and the proposal offered credible options that would draw the attention of the administration to explore these issues.

There is no guarantee of the outcome, but the discussion between José and his administrative leader maintained integrity, reflected the team's values, and respected the values of the clinic. Using the decision-making matrix offered a process to lead José to this proposal under consideration.

Challenges to Ethics

Today's social and political culture presents challenges to personal ethics. Deeply held values and morals of the leader may not meet with the approval of current societal norms. The APP leader may find sincere team members in disagreement with his or her personally held values and should be prepared to hold discussions in respect to differing values:

» **Scientific reasoning is not paramount:** The most reasoned evidence is not necessarily convincing to the team if it is still in conflict with personally held values.

» **Morality and truth are not absolute:** Others do not necessarily patently agree with what the leader considers true or moral.

» **Hypocrisy prevents reliable reasoning:** Attempts to support values and morals on sound behavior are pointed out as ineffective because of the moral failings of some leaders as noted by others.

» **Authority is removed in the name of tolerance:** There is no such thing as preeminent authority, so ascribing to a high authority without a more reasoned basis is thought to be boorish and presumptive.

While the challenges of these perspectives may add conflict, recognizing these as socially acceptable disagreements guides the APP leader to navigate the future course. The team may not tacitly accept leader decisions based solely on absolute truth, scientific reasoning, or an esteemed authority figure.

Ethical Integrity

Definitions of integrity are consistently about honesty and virtues. The leader who acts with integrity is then sincere in upholding high moral behavior. In today's environment, unethical behaviors strain to appear legitimate. Scandals in leadership are common occurrences. The APP leader who stands above the fray, striving to maintain personal integrity, will earn the respect of the team. Consistently speaking with honesty and candor with the team, staying true to commitments, taking responsibility for all actions, and owning mistakes while correcting them, all build an ethical leader. When the more severe challenges arise, responding with these attributes by conscientious and compassionate means helps maintain integrity above reproach.

CROSSING CULTURE

Today, the APP need only look across the waiting room to explore culture. Most APP graduates from this millennium have been exposed to the Institute of Medicine (IOM) report *Unequal Treatment: Confronting Racial/ Ethnic Disparities in Health Care*, documenting over 175 studies of racial/ ethnic health disparities in the diagnosis and treatment of often common conditions (2003). In response, an evidence-based conceptual model of cultural competence was presented to overcome the sociocultural barriers that prevented care across all racial and ethnic populations (Betancourt, Green, Carrilla, & Ananeh-Firempong II, 2003)

Near the same time as the IOM's report, the Association of American Medical Colleges (AAMC) brought forth a clarion call to train the next generation of physicians to be "culturally competent." A well-developed curriculum was presented with tools for measuring competency across five domains:

» **Domain I:** Cultural Competence Rationale, Context and Definition

» **Domain II:** Key Aspects of Cultural Competence

» **Domain III:** Understanding the Impact of Stereotyping on Medical Decision Making

» **Domain IV:** Health Disparities and Factors Influencing Health

» **Domain V:** Cross-Cultural Clinical Skills

In the AAMC publication, *Cultural Competency Education for Medical Students* (2005), culture is defined as "the integrated pattern of human behavior that includes language, thoughts, customs, beliefs, and institutions of racial, ethnic, social or religious groups" (Cross, Bazron, Dennis, & Isaacs, 1989). This is an inclusive definition that engages all people in discussions of culture. While overt hallmarks of culture may indicate age, ethnic heritage, or country of origin (e.g., behavior, dress, language, and diet), discussions of culture in health care include issues of gender, sexual orientation, and religion that may not be as noticeable.

The AAMC's elaborate curriculum teaches awareness, knowledge, and skills needed by health professionals to recognize and respond to distinctions of culture related to health and disease. Evaluation measures for medical students involved over 70 elements of attitudes, knowledge, and skills across the five domains. Students accomplish these learning goals of competency in their preclinical studies and again in their clinical clerkships. Success over these measures indicates reaching a standard of cultural competency.

CULTURALLY INFORMED

While the pursuit of cultural competence among health care professionals remains common language, more sociologists and others are using the term "culturally informed" to suggest a continuum of growth (Kleinman & Benson, 2006). Developing culturally informed health care professionals avoids a set of standards to achieve to be competent. Rather, health care professionals consider their awareness of culture and are encouraged to do what is necessary to advance toward greater cultural awareness, knowledge, and skills.

Becoming culturally informed, then, describes a process rather than an endpoint, fostering a continual growth of cultural development over a life span. *Intercultural sensitivity* is the goal, a growing ability to distinguish and experience various cultural influences (Bennett, 1986). As society becomes more culturally blended by immigrant and migrant influx, workforce population shifts and the relative ease of international exchange, APPs must join all health professionals in developing intercultural sensitivity.

In a thoughtful approach to cultural development, the first step for APP leaders is to self-determine one's position on a continuum from ethnocentricism (one's own culture is central to others) to ethnorelativism (cultures are understood in relation to another without priority). Three stages of development are associated with each pole of this continuum (Bennett, 1986).

Stages of Ethnocentricism

Stage 1 – Denial: There is only one culture so there are no cultural differences.
Stage 2 – Defense/Reversal: Two opposing ideals represent this stage, based on there being one dominant culture superior to all others. Either an individual holds to that culture (defense) or holds to another culture one believes as inferior to the dominant culture (reversal).
Stage 3 – Minimization: Since all humans are biologically the same, there is no distinction of different cultures.

Stages of Ethnorelativism

Stage 4 – Acceptance: One's own culture is understood to be among other equally complex worldviews.
Stage 5 – Adaptation: Engaging other cultures requires a perspective within the context of each culture. This stage can be divided into cognitive (knowledge of cultures) and behavioral (interactions with cultures) categories.
Stage 6 – Integration: Fully aware of one's own culture, appreciation and value is shared between cultures.

An honest self-reflection by an APP leader reveals where he or she falls on this continuum (see Figure 9.1). If a more formal process is desired, the Intercultural Development Inventory (IDI) is a 50-item survey instrument developed to establish the position of an individual among these six stages (Hammer, Bennett, & Wiseman, 2003). The administration of the IDI requires a trained examiner.

A common outcome of the IDI when administered in Western cultures finds individuals at the minimization stage. That stage most avoids the complexities of different cultures by a universal characterization that all humans are basically the same. Culture viewed in this way has been commonly taught in primary and secondary U.S. schools over recent generations. Minimization is a developmental advance from the denial and defense/reversal stages, but it remains ethnocentric, as it does not value the distinctions of different cultures.

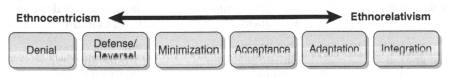

FIGURE 9.1 Stages of intercultural development.
Source: Adapted from Bennett (1986).

Intercultural Sensitivity and APP Leadership

Matkin and Barbuto (2012) explored relationships between Leader-Member Exchange (LMX) theory (see Chapter 5) and intercultural sensitivity. Their study measured LMX ratings compared to the IDI assessment in 72 leaders and 255 followers in higher education. Leaders with a higher level of intercultural sensitivity had a higher follower rating of LMX. Of interest, variables of gender, race, or sexual orientation did not predict LMX ratings of the leader. For example, a high level of intercultural sensitivity was positively related to a high follower rating, but indication of gender, race, or sexual orientation of the leader did not correlate with a high follower rating in this study.

Applying this to APP leaders, team members may respond positively in the LMX relationship with the leader if growth in intercultural sensitivity is noted in the leader. In the multicultural environments of most health care delivery systems, it is important for APP leaders to advance in cultural development. The leader may also benefit from evaluating the level of intercultural sensitivity of the team. In the health care environment, the APP leader will find value in sponsoring activities for the team that foster growth in intercultural sensitivity. Table 9.2 offers activities the leader can institute to help advance team members along the continuum toward ethnorelativism.

TABLE 9.2 Activities to Advance Stages of Intercultural Development

Intercultural Sensitivity Shift	Goal	Activity
From defense/reversal to minimization	Identify characteristics of nondominant cultures	Celebrating holidays, enjoying cultural foods, other exposures to differences in culture
From minimization to acceptance	Find value in distinctions of nondominant cultures	Hosting speakers or workshops on different cultures
From acceptance to adaptation	Engage others to experience cultural distinctions	Relational activities, pairing individuals from different cultures
From adaption to integration	Able to smoothly transfer between cultures	Immersing oneself in a different culture by fieldtrip or other cultural travels

Implicit Leadership Theory and APPs

Obstacles to cultural development are expected as a part of the journey and, when recognized, help develop one to be more culturally informed. Among the obstacles APP leaders may face are misperceptions from team members regarding issues of culture. Such assumptions are not always correct. In the common roles of mentoring among health care professionals, influences can be subtle in communication about dress, tastes, opinions, mannerisms, and judgments.

All clinicians are cued by individual socialization to view and value people in certain ways (Wear, Kumagai, Varley, & Zarconi (2012). Referring to the "Gall bladder in room 3" is one common example of mistakenly calling a patient with gall bladder disease only by the name of the organ. Others' perceptions may find that such language diminishes an appreciation for the patient's holistic qualities as a person. The leader should be alert to the team misperceiving her or his intentions and use such opportunities to explore different perspectives and cultural values, fostering open discussions.

The Implicit Leadership Theory (Offermann, Kennedy, & Wirtz, 1994) refers to how groups will have implicit perceptions about the leader, often related to personal and inherent characteristics of the leader. These perceptions (termed "ILTs") create a framework through which team members interpret all other information about the leader.

For example, if the APP leader is viewed as consistently wearing expensive clothing, the ILTs may lead the team to assume that the APP is pretentious about appearance. While no mention is made, his or her attire may consistently reinforce this attitude toward the APP. Later this may create a commotion when asking the APP to volunteer at a local homeless shelter. Some may suggest that the APP would not be interested or willing to volunteer because of the implicit leader assumptions (that the APP is too consumed with expensive tastes to consider working in a homeless shelter) deeply held around the team for perhaps months or years.

In the LMX/IDI study by Matkin & Barbuto discussed earlier, the implicit leadership theory supports why a team would have higher LMX scores for the leader who has a higher level of intercultural sensitivity. The team recognizes the leader's commitment to advancing in ethorelativism.

The APP leader should recognize that team members are actively but implicitly making these assumptions. If leadership is waning, it may indicate that there are undesirable perceptions among the team that deserve exploration and response.

APP Lessons From the GLOBE Study

A comprehensive and ongoing study of leadership styles and cultural perceptions, including 62 different cultures, is the Global Leadership and

Organizational Behavior Effectiveness (GLOBE) Study, approaching its third decade of work. The extensive results and outcomes, shared in a significant report in 2004 (House, Hanges, Javidan, Dorfman, & Gupta, 2004), continue to inform leadership in organizational cultures across the world. APPs who have the pleasure and privilege of serving with multicultural teams will find the constructs derived from the GLOBE study of help in understanding variations of culture in reference to leadership.

VARIATIONS IN THE IDEAL LEADER

Based on culturally endorsed implicit leadership theory principles, nine dimensions of value distinctions between cultures were identified and measured as opposite poles (i.e., high or low). Six of these value dimensions are selected for exploration by APP leaders here: performance orientation, humane orientation, power distance, uncertainty avoidance, gender egalitarianism, and individualism/collectivism (see Table 9.3).

TABLE 9.3 Value Dimensions Across Cultures

Value Dimension	High	Low
Performance orientation	Ethic of hard work, achievement-oriented, competitive	Status based on position, entitlements; achievements less important
Humane orientation	Concern for others on team, self-sacrificing	More autocratic and utilitarian; less personalized
Power distance	Leaders with authority, team is compliant, rules and policies enforced	Less rigid structure; team participates in leadership
Uncertainty avoidance	Team fears the unknown and expects stability, security, order	Team accepts uncertainty and disorder; more flexible and willing to take risks
Gender egalitarianism	Gender roles are indistinguishable	Masculine and feminine attributes are distinguished
Individualism/ collectivism*	Individualism emphasizes personal interests and goals of team members	Collectivism emphasizes goals of group over individual interests

*The spectrum of this value dimension is not from high to low, but from individualism to collectivism.

» **Performance orientation:** High performance orientation in a leader includes attributes of hard work, initiative, and competitiveness. Results are emphasized more than people so that achievements are an important source of status. Low performance orientation emphasizes entitlements to individuals based on their position rather than achievements.

» **Humane orientation:** High humane orientation indicates a leader with great concern for the welfare of others, represented by altruistic and benevolent behaviors. Low humane orientation is more autocratic, with leader skills representing utilitarian attributes (decisions based on the greatest good for the greatest number).

» **Power distance:** In high power distance, leaders are granted great authority and the team is compliant, following rules with functional policies in force. In low power distance, the leadership hierarchy is less rigid. The leader role may be more ambiguous with shared leadership.

» **Uncertainty avoidance:** High uncertainty avoidance indicates a culture that fears the unknown so the team is dependent on stability, security, and order. In low uncertainty avoidance, the team accepts disorder, so the leader can be more flexible and take risks.

» **Gender egalitarianism:** Egalitarianism refers to the equal treatment of all, so this value dimension measures if gender roles are distinguished. In high gender egalitarianism, there is little differentiation of gender roles. In low gender egalitarianism, masculine roles (identified as more autocratic, harsh, assertive) are distinguished from feminine roles (identified as more relational, compassionate, intuitive).

This value dimension is not a measure of gender discrimination, which holds no place in the roles of APPs. There is no empirical support that either gender is more qualified than the other, and laws exist in the United States to prevent sex-based discrimination.

» **Individualism/Collectivism:** In an individualism value dimension, autonomy is a priority; the personal interests and goals of each team member are emphasized. In collectivistic cultures, the goals of the group have priority over individual interests. Loyalty to the group's interests is emphasized.

While these value dimensions help the APP leader consider perspectives from team members who may have a cultural view distinct from the leader's own, there is much overlap in these dimensions. It is difficult to assign one dimension to a particular people group or culture. For example, an individual may have high power distance (leaders with authority over compliant team) and high humane orientation (concern for the team's welfare), but how much influence each value holds may vary.

APPs Leading Across Cultures

Data from the GLOBE Study (Dorfman, Hanges, & Brodbeck, 2004) have also contributed to determining which leader attributes are effective across most cultures, compared to attributes that may vary in effectiveness in different cultures. Those leadership traits with high effectiveness across cultures that align with the APP leader include leaders who are visionary, decisive, dynamic, dependable, encouraging, and excellence oriented. The list also includes the trait of honesty, skills in administration, and effectiveness in integrating teams.

Attributes that may differ among cultures may deserve individual attention by the APP leader. For example, the ambitious leader may be well suited in some cultures, but less welcomed in others. APPs working in multicultural environments should take notice of these attributes that may vary across cultures, including the cautious, compassionate, or humble leader—while the character trait is admirable, the leadership attribute may lead to implicit assumptions or misperceptions among the team.

LEADING MILLENIALS

The largest living generation in the United States is now Millennials, surpassing Baby Boomers in 2016 (Fry, 2016). With this comes a generation with different expectations of leaders. In concluding this chapter on ethics and culture, exploring the characteristics of this generation offers a summative review of the concepts explored.

While some are quick to identify contrary attitudes among Millennials (those born between 1980 and 2000), as a group they are the most diverse, best educated (though the majority are undereducated), and most intentionally reared generation of the times. In light of implicit leadership theory and cultural distinctions, the APP who is leading Millennials on the health care team may find the following recommendations useful.

» **Offer an ethical team:** Millennials are concerned about social responsibility and seek membership with an organization that practices high ethical standards. The APP leader should ensure that the team's integrity is upheld and above reproach.

» **Shared obligation:** Millennials are accused of being overly entitled. What appears to be a lack of taking responsibility and working hard is actually a participative desire to have responsibilities distributed across a team, which breeds success.

» **Give balance:** Learning a lesson from their overachieving Baby Boomer parents, Millennials avoid lifestyle choices that put their personal lives out of balance with work. APP leaders champion this cause with

Millennials, creating reasonable work schedules and balancing on-call responsibilities with time off.

» **Provide feedback:** The implicit assumption is that Millennials avoid working independently. However, they are rather seeking feedback to be sure their work has the desired impact. Regular, informal advice with constructive criticism (e.g., following surgical procedures or patient evaluations) will likely foster a stronger work ethic and reach anticipated outcomes.

EXERCISE 9.1 MINDFUL STEREOTYPING

Relying on rigid, deeply engrained categories (e.g., old/young, masculine/feminine, White/non-White) supports implicit assumptions that lead to mindless stereotyping (Ting-Toomey, 1999). To counteract this tendency, exploring mindful stereotyping *broadens one's worldview and may correct misperceptions and unintentional prejudice.*

1. *Select an activity that engages an individual or group with a different culture (e.g., enjoying a meal at an ethnic restaurant, attending a holiday celebration, or visiting a home, event, or fair that represents another culture).*

2. *Reflect beforehand on any expectations held, such as if it will be enjoyable, how much time it will take, intentions on doing this multiple times or just once, and so on, and recognize any anxieties.*

3. *At the activity, use all senses to note distinctions that may reflect different cultures (e.g., eye-to-eye contact with others, odors and aromas, languages spoken, music, spices and flavorings of food, textures and colors of dress). Use the ODIS model in considering these distinctions: Observe, Describe, Interpret, and Suspend evaluation.*

4. *During any social interaction with another person (e.g., the host, the waitress/waiter, and other guests), quickly come up with two or three ideas of what the person likes mentally (e.g., favorite athletic teams, media shows, food, and hobbies). Then while visiting, ask the person to tell you their favorites. Compare answers.*

5. *After the activity, self-reflect on the expectations identified in item 2. Engage in a discussion with a trusted friend to explore your own openness to new information, your ability to make correct assumptions, and any context of the culture that is newly recognized. Identify any prior categorizations that have now changed or expanded.*

SUMMARY POINTS

1. The practice of leadership by APPs benefits from following the same ethical principles that guide clinical practice: nonmaleficience, patient autonomy, beneficence, and justice. Ethical dilemmas that leaders face should be processed through the decision-making matrix that includes these principles. In more challenging dilemmas, the principles of non-maleficence and autonomy may give greater guidance.

2. In today's social culture, there is greater diversity of values and view-points that bring disagreements within health care teams. As debates arise from disagreements in personally held values among the team members, the APP may be able to lead a discussion that keeps the team moving forward while respecting different viewpoints. When faced with team conflict, the leader should act with integrity by listening well, speaking with honesty, and honoring commitments.

3. All health care professionals are expected to grow in their understanding of the cultural implications in medicine. Becoming culturally informed is a continual process that yields greater intercultural sensitivity. APPs should recognize their own awareness of culture and develop themselves across the stages of minimization (the final stage of ethnocentricism) to acceptance, adaptation and integration (all stages of ethnorelativism). As they become self-aware of intercultural sensitivity, leaders can help the team also advance toward ethnorelativism.

4. The path of cultural development holds challenges for the leader, as team members will make assumptions that can be unfounded and interfere with progress. Unintentional behaviors leave cues that are misinterpreted by others and lead to implicit perceptions that may be undiscovered until a challenge or conflict occurs. The APP leader who practices mindful awareness of potential differences in cultural perceptions (i.e., performance orientation, human orientation, power distance, uncertainty avoidance, gender egalitarianism, and individu-alism/collectivism) is positioned to discover and respond to unspoken assumptions that need correction.

REFERENCES

Association of American Medical Colleges. (2005). *Cultural Competence Education for Medical Students*. Washington, DC: Author.

Bennett, J. M. (1986). A developmental approach to training for intercultural sensitivity. *International Journal of Intercultural Relations, 10*(2), 79–95.

Betancourt, J. R., Green, A. R., Carrilla, J. E., & Ananeh-Firempong, O., II. (2003). Defining cultural competence: A practical framework for addressing racial/ethnic disparities in health and health care. *Public Health Reports, 118*, 293–302.

Cross, T. L., Bazron, B. J., Dennis, K. W., & Isaacs, M. R. (1989). *Toward a culturally competent system of care: A monograph on effective services for minority children who are severely emotionally disturbed.* Washington, DC: Georgetown University.

Dorfman, P. W., Hanges, P. J., & Brodbeck, F. C. (2004). Leadership and cultural variation: Identification of culturally endorsed leadership profiles. In R. J. House, P. J. Hanges, M. Javidan, P. W. Dorfman, & V. Gupta (Eds.), *Culture, leadership, and organizations: The GLOBE study of 62 societies* (pp. 669–719), Thousand Oaks, CA: Sage.

Fry, R. (2016). Millennials overtake Baby Boomers as America's largest generation. *Fact Tank.* Retrieved from http://pewrsr.ch/1UcT1B3

Hammer, M. R., Bennett, M. J., & Wiseman, R. (2003). Measuring intercultural sensitivity: The intercultural development inventory. *International Journal of Intercultural Relations, 27*, 421–444.

House, R. J., Hanges, P. J., Javidan, M., Dorfman, P. W., & Gupta, V. (Eds.) (2004). *Culture, leadership, and organizations: The GLOBE study of 62 societies.* Thousand Oaks, CA: Sage.

Jonsen, A. R., Siegler, M., & Winsalde, W. J. (2015). *Clinical ethics: A practical approach to ethical decisions in clinical medicine* (8th ed.). New York, NY: McGraw-Hill.

Kaldjian, L. C., Weir, R. F., & Duffy, T. P. (2005). A clinician's approach to clinical ethics. *Journal of General Internal Medicine, 20*(3), 306–3011.

Kleinman, A., & Benson, P. (2006). Anthropology in the clinic: The problem of cultural competency and how to fix it. *PLOS Medicine, 3*(10), e294. doi:10.1371/journal.pmed.0030294

Matkin, G. S., & Barbuto, J. E. (2012). Demographic similarity/difference, intercultural sensitivity, and leader-member exchange: A multilevel analysis. *Journal of Leadership & Organizational Studies, 19*(3), 294–302.

Offermann, L. R., Kennedy, J. K., & Wirtz, P. W. (1994). Implicit leadership theories: Content, structure, and generalizability. *The Leadership Quarterly, 5*(1), 43–58.

Ting-Toomey, S. (1999). *Communication across cultures* (pp. 163–164). New York, NY: Guilford Press.

Wear, D., Kumagai, A. K., Varley, J., & Zarconi, J. (2012). Cultural competency 2.0: Exploring the concept of difference in engagement with the other. *Academic Medicine, 87*(6), 1–7.

Yukl, G. (2013). *Leadership in organizations* (8th ed.). Upper Saddle River, NJ: Pearson.

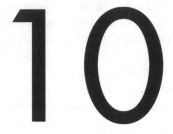

10
QUALITIES OF SPIRITUAL LEADERSHIP IN A CLINICAL SETTING

CRITICAL THINKING QUESTIONS

» **Do spiritual leadership principles apply to advanced practice providers (APPs) in health care settings?**

» **What spiritual leadership skills are effective in leading others in health care delivery?**

» **Is there a way to measure spiritual well-being in health care teams?**

Spiritual leadership is rooted in intrinsic motivations that guide the leader to cast vision and convey hope in behaviors representing altruistic love (Fry, 2003). When applied to the workplace, spirituality is distinguished from religion and is broadly inclusive of two perceived human needs—to *be called* to a purpose and to *belong* to a group (Fry, 2003). To avoid confusion, spirituality used here is separate from religion so that there is no implied or obvious support for any specific theological or religious leanings.

The APP may not initially see the value of spiritual leadership if the individual is not "spiritual" or comfortable in exploring what may feel like more intimate, personal ideologies. However, the APP leader should recognize that there is a transcendent drive in every human being that in various ways represents a calling to a purpose and having membership with others. Spiritual leadership skills are helpful to address this internal drive, directed toward the group of team members as well as to an individual, such as when caring for a patient. These concepts deserve further study regarding the terms used and associated behaviors.

CASE STUDY 1

Regina was at her desk finishing patient records at the end of a long shift working as an APP at the local hospital emergency department when she was interrupted.

"Got a minute?" Nathan, an APP colleague, asked at the doorway to her office.

"Sure, come on in," Regina responded and gestured for him to sit in a nearby chair. "What's up?"

"I'm just wondering," Nathan took a deep breath before continuing, "maybe I'm not cut out for this."

"What do you mean?" Regina asked. "Having a bad day?"

Regina had held this position for over a decade and had helped recruit Nathan, who started 3 years ago. She had oriented him to the position and continued to advise him in his role.

"Not just a bad day," he responded, dejectedly. "But you . . . you seem to roll with things."

"It's about the copycat suicides, isn't it?" Regina offered. The community had suffered three teen suicides in the past month, the last two clearly triggered by the first one. She knew Nathan had been on-call when the last one was brought in.

"Maybe that's a part of it," Nathan said, "but I've been thinking about this for a while now. I just don't bounce back like you do when things are tough around here. It makes me wonder if there might be a better spot for me."

Nathan was clearly serious, and he saw Regina as his mentor. How she responds to his vulnerable request for help has the potential to change lives.

No leader feels prepared for every single challenge ahead. Successful leaders likely are those who are responsive to change and able to adapt to new situations, bringing the team along. Those traits are noticed and admired by others, which leads to new leadership opportunities. It also garners the respect of others, which brings occasions like Regina has in Case Study 1, the opportunity to shape a life. The wise leader will pause to fully consider the most meaningful response.

As voiced by Nathan, the need to feel called to a life of meaning and purpose and the need to feel a part of something (membership) are deeply rooted human needs. His internal, or intrinsic, motivation to serve patients in this environment is in question. Regina may seek to draw on spiritual leadership skills to help Nathan resolve his personal dilemma.

INTRINSIC MOTIVATION

Traditional models of motivation do not sufficiently explain the diversity of behaviors observed in the workplace. The general premise that people function best in their occupation through the anticipation of achieving goals and rewards does not provide occupational satisfaction among most professionals. While these motivations have their place, neglecting intrinsic motivation leads to ultimate dissatisfaction.

Maslow (1943) explored the five-step hierarchy of needs that intimated global, intrinsic sources of motivation:

1. **Physiological:** Basic needs of existence (e.g., hunger and thirst)

2. **Safety:** Need for security

3. **Love:** Need for affection and belonging

4. **Esteem:** Need for self-respect and respect from others

5. **Self-actualization:** Pursuing the full potential of what a person could become

Alderfer (1969) reduced Maslow's hierarchy of five needs into three:

» **Existence:** Physiological and safety

» **Relatedness:** Esteem and love

» **Growth:** Self-actualization

This ERG theory suggested that motivations are all internal and they overlap, compensating for another need at each level if necessary.

By reinterpreting previous research, Ryan and Deci (2000) developed the self-determination theory (SDT) to explore the continuum of motivation (see Figure 10.1). At one end is the amotivated person with no self-determination—a person who does not act at all, or is simply going through the motions due to having no value assigned to the activity, having no sense of competence, or having no expectation of a desired outcome. At the opposite end is a pure state of intrinsic motivation, a fully self-determined behavior that a person does for no apparent reward except the activity itself or the feelings that result from the activity.

In the middle of the continuum are four classifications of decreasing levels of extrinsic motivation (e.g., the external demands or rewards that provide incentives). The fourth level, nearest to the most complete state of intrinsic motivation, represents a point when external motivation is purely

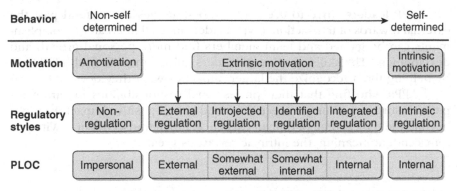

FIGURE 10.1 The self-determination theory.
PLOC, perceived locus of control.
Source: Slightly modified from Ryan and Deci (2000).

congruent with the person's personal values (integrated regulation). It is at this point that the professional realistically finds the greatest satisfaction in his or her actions.

By definition, spiritual leadership comprises the values, attitudes, and behaviors necessary to intrinsically motivate the leader and those influenced by the leader with a sense of calling and membership (Fry, 2003). Leaders who inspire their team by appealing to this intrinsic motivation that meets these human needs will practice spiritual leadership.

LEADERSHIP AND INTRINSIC MOTIVATION

Several of the leadership models described in this text focus on the leader motivating the health care team, including path–goal, charismatic, servant, adaptive, and transformation leadership. Kouzes and Posner (2012), who have for over 30 years researched and explored their *Five Practices of Exemplary Leadership*, identify each leadership behavior founded in intrinsic motivation:

> » **Model the way:** Affirm shared values and set the example

> » **Inspire a shared vision:** Appeal to shared aspirations

> » **Challenge the process:** Take risks and learn from experience

> » **Enable others to act:** Build trust and strengthen others to develop competence

> » **Encourage the art:** Show appreciation for others and celebrate victories

APP leaders strive to use leadership strategies that extend past the external rewards of transactional-type leadership so that greater accomplishments can be gained and team members find more personal growth and development. The skills of spiritual leaders guide others to find fulfillment by helping them recognize the larger impact of what they do.

APPs who find that their professional responsibilities in caring for patients surpass ordinary expectations and have a positive impact that goes beyond the typical drag of human existence, touch transcendence. With this transcendent meaning, the intrinsic reward is great.

CASE STUDY 1 (*CONTINUED*)

"So Nathan, what brings you to this point of questioning your abilities?" *Regina asked.*

"I just don't feel like I'm making a difference," Nathan answered. "Too often what I'm doing is relieving a headache that's only going to come back, or getting a drug abuser dried out only to return next week. It's hard to believe that's much help. How do you find doing this rewarding?"

TRANSCENDENT MEANING AND SPIRITUALITY

Robert Greenleaf, in writing about servant leadership, suggested the test of this leadership in answering the following questions:

> Do those served grow as persons? Do they, while being served, become healthier, wiser, freer, more autonomous, more likely themselves to become servants? And what is the effect on the least privileged in society; will they benefit, or at least, not be further deprived? (Greenleaf, 1977, p. 24)

By this measure of outcomes, positive answers indicate if the result is better than predicted, exceeding common expectations. In health care, it would not only measure if the APP is able to alleviate disease in patients, but more so identify if the APP is able to help patients improve their health, bringing opportunities for those patients to have a greater positive effect on others and society. An APP who is aware of influencing others to this end will experience a transcendent internal reward. In Case Study 1, this is what Nathan is missing.

This transcendent meaning is grounded in a commitment to high virtues, including compassion, humility, integrity, gratitude, forgiveness, trust, and loyalty. The leader, by actions more than words, demonstrates a consistent practice of virtues that draws others to do the same. Spirituality draws this transcendent meaning in two domains: life scheme and self-efficacy.

» **Life scheme:** Personal satisfaction with life, life purpose, and positive and negative life experiences are critical components of existential well-being (Diener, 2000). This personal view of a meaningful life is a measurable mediator to well-being (Wong, 1998). These measurable elements include factors of relationship, achievement, and self-transcendence, in parallel with the human spiritual need for membership and a call to purpose.

» **Self-efficacy:** Described as an individual's belief in the capacity to organize and perform tasks necessary to achieve a goal (Bandura, 1997), self-efficacy operationalizes a person's functionality in his or her life scheme. Several studies have shown a positive correlation between job involvement and self-efficacy. Donnay and Borgen (1999) found self-efficacy as a valid and distinct measure of occupational satisfaction among 21 different occupational groups, ranging from farmers to auto mechanics to architects to teachers.

Spiritual Well-Being

Combining a person's life scheme (personal satisfaction with life) and self-efficacy (belief in one's own ability to perform) suggests a measure of spiritual well-being (Daaleman, Cobb, & Frey, 2001).

A study of physicians revealed that of the four dimensions of satisfaction (personal, professional, inherent, and performance), the most important dimension for all specialties and patterns of practice was inherent satisfaction (Lepnurm, Danielson, Dobson, & Keegan, 2006). The study concluded that these higher-order needs of satisfaction are important to motivate superior performance in clinical and nonclinical tasks, again suggesting that life scheme and self-efficacy are interrelated.

Therefore, awareness of one's personal life scheme and self-efficacy provides a sense of one's spiritual well-being. That self-awareness positions the individual to be able to lead spiritually. The same process applied to the others on that leader's team may guide opportunities to help others in spiritual well-being.

John Maxwell (2011), a former pastor who later led a leadership training company that boasts training 5 million leaders worldwide and has had several bestseller books selling well over 20 million copies, writes that there are five levels of leadership: (a) position, (b) permission, (c) production, (d) people development, and (e) pinnacle. The lowest level (position) is based on the title assigned to the leader. The second level (permission) indicates others want to follow the leader and the third level (production) indicates the team is getting things done under the leader. He suggests that effective leaders grow to the more advanced levels by first helping other leaders at level 4 (people development), and lastly to level 5 (pinnacle) by developing other leaders to level 4. In his own words, "You see, my passion in life is growing and equipping others to do remarkable things and lead significant and fulfilled lives." By his own example and his leadership training, he helps others develop a meaningful life scheme with high self-efficacy, meeting the calling of a spiritual leader.

LIMITATIONS OF SPIRITUAL LEADERSHIP

There is a clear association between individuals who practice consistent spiritual values and their effectiveness as leaders (Reave, 2005). However, the wide mix of values associated with spirituality prevents a defined construct specific for spiritual leadership. The processes by which leaders influence others defy a consistent explanation. It is then difficult to determine how one becomes a spiritual leader (Yukl, 2013).

This leaves much of the writing on spiritual leadership to conjecture, true in this chapter as well. A connection between spirituality and effective leadership is evident so that exploring it in the context of APPs in the health care environment deserves attention.

BEHAVIORS OF THE SPIRITUAL LEADER

Behaviors common to the spiritual leader are casting vision, conveying hope, and practicing altruistic love. The positive correlation of these types of qualities and effective leadership is clear (Fry, 2003).

Casting Vision

Developing a vision for an individual or a team cannot follow a mechanical formula, as analysis and judgment are required. An appealing vision represents a high degree of intuition and creativity. Four characteristics of an effective vision include:

» ***Clarity:*** A clear reason for the directive must be defendable. When inevitable questions and doubts arise, the vision should give clarity to refocus the team.

» ***Idealistic:*** The appeal of the vision must reach toward a goal that is unquestionably desirable.

» ***Challenging:*** The vision is expected to be daunting, requiring extra—if not extraordinary—effort while being realistic.

» ***Attainable:*** The path may not be clear, but it is conceivable, not fantasy.

All key stakeholders must participate in creating an effective vision. A single leader needs the collective wisdom of the group to consider all implications.

Conveying Hope

When uncertainty exists, a loss of the team's direction is predictable, and scattered wandering is next. Returning to the expectation that something of great benefit is ahead conveys hope. Absolute certainty is not the objective. Expressing hope that the purpose or mission of the effort is yet worth pursuing keeps the team together.

Conveying hope reinforces the sense of calling, that life has meaning. Communicating hope by reviewing the elements of an effective vision, reestablishing the clearly challenging but attainable ideal, keeps the team's direction focused and moving forward.

Practicing Altruistic Love

Altruism has been described as a stage of human development or a modeled behavior, but it remains difficult to define by a measure. An altruistic act is pro-social, coming from an internal motivation that holds no external benefit or tangible reward to self. Altruism is directly associated with spirituality as it brings a transcendent connection between the selfless action and the benefit to others. A relationship between altruism and a healthy mental state exists, with altruistic actions supporting one's desirable self-esteem. Lastly, and most importantly, explanations of altruism are not complete without an understanding of the motivation of love (Mastain, 2006).

Love, in this context, is the sincere appreciation and expressed valuing of the well-being of oneself or others. Altruistic love is then a sense of harmony and completeness emanating from the care, concern, and appreciation for self and others. Achieving altruistic love is subjective and not quantifiable, but few would argue that it is never completely reached. Therefore, altruistic love is practiced, a goal to strive for.

An Example: Clara Barton

The qualities ascribed to spiritual leadership can be daunting, setting a standard of unrealistic perfection. Spiritual leadership challenges the APP in effectively applying these skills of casting vision, conveying hope, and practicing altruistic love.

Clara Barton (1821–1912) offers a historical example from which to learn, as told by D. A. Forrester in *Nursing's Greatest Leaders* (2016). During the Civil War, before any nursing education programs were established in the United States, Clara Barton willingly traveled the battlefields to care for the injured and comfort the dying, earning her a reputation for heroic exploits at the frontlines of combat. Later she volunteered to manage the records of soldiers reported as "missing," with President Abraham Lincoln personally directing the public to her services. Her humanitarian efforts led her to the International Red Cross, and she learned the U.S. government had yet to sign an agreement to support efforts to care for wartime soldiers (already established by the Treaty of Geneva in 1864, signed by 11 countries). Barton began a movement through the presidential administrations of Lincoln, Hayes, and Garfield, until finally President Arthur signed the treaty in 1882. One year prior to that, Barton was named the inaugural president of the Red Cross Society, continuing to lead the organization for 23 years in what is now recognized as the American Red Cross.

Clara Barton sustained herself and her supporters with consistent vision, hope, and altruism. To understand her full character of leadership, it is important to recognize that her record was not unblemished. There were reports of embellished war stories, a brief affair, flawed financial accounting, questions of her mental health, and an independent spirit that occasionally raised controversy. Despite this, Barton's life holds a reputation for great courage and tireless work in leading the cause of bringing humanitarian aid to those in need.

Returning to this chapter's case study brings a current-day example where these same skills of spiritual leadership are useful.

CASE STUDY 1 (*CONTINUED*)

"Don't kid yourself, Nathan, I have my bad days," Regina said. "You're going through a tough season. I know you're wrestling with the deaths of those recent suicides. We all are, but it hit deep with you."

"That was rough," Nathan responded quietly. "I felt so helpless, and that boy I took care of . . . had his whole life ahead of him."

"So we lost that one," Regina said. "And we mourn and cry if we need to. But tomorrow there's someone else who needs you."

Nathan objected, staring at the floor. "I'm not sure I want to try again tomorrow."

"I get it, and it's the way I feel, too, sometimes. But I don't know when that next headache or sniffle is actually someone who might be on the brink of suicide. Maybe that's the one I can do something about."

Nathan raised his eyes to meet Regina's.

"That's why I'll be here tomorrow, Nathan. I hope you'll be here, too."

RESULTS OF SPIRITUAL LEADERSHIP

Whether Regina knew it or not, she was using spiritual leadership skills with Nathan in Case Study 1. Nathan had lost his calling and didn't feel like he belonged. By what Regina said, speaking of her own values though she knew they were shared with him, she was able to touch Nathan's deepest felt needs.

Calling: Nathan has lost his resolve to care for others. Regina reminds him that caring for the patient with simple complaints may actually be helping more deeply than he knows, even perhaps preventing a suicide tendency from rising.

Membership: Nathan does not feel like he belongs in the ER with Regina. She makes it clear that she wants him to come back.

In Nathan's situation, addressing his deep needs of calling and membership will likely help re-center his own life scheme and self-efficacy. Regina has shared with him her vision for her own work in the ER, identified that while it is challenging, it is attainable. Her vision also conveys a hope that her actions (and his) may possibly save a life (idealistic).

Lastly, her compassion shows as altruistic love. In positive psychology, altruistic love overcomes destructive influences such as fear (including anxiety), anger (including resentment), a sense of failure (including self-destructive guilt), and selfishness (including conceit) (Seligman & Csikszentmihalyi, 2000).

All principles of spiritual leadership are reflected in Regina's discussion with Nathan and it provides a model for how APP leaders can use these skills in helping the team around them.

SPIRITUAL WELL-BEING

In this chapter's case study, Nathan raised his concerns directly to Regina, and she wisely recognized the need for renewing his sense of calling and membership. If Nathan had not directly approached Regina, she may not have known the frustrations he was facing. This is common to the challenge of identifying the sound well-being of others on the team. The leader must be vigilant to identify cues that indicate an individual is discouraged or wrestling with these issues. Measures of spiritual well-being can indicate the level of personal satisfaction that individuals hold in themselves.

Nearly a thousand nurse practitioners (NPs) and physician assistants (PAs) were polled on the level of job satisfaction, with results published in the December 2016 *Clinician Reviews*. Of the projectable sample size, 63% were NPs and 34.1% were PAs (4.6% marked "other" to indicate research, academic, etc.). Asked if given the chance to do it again, 85% responded they would choose the same career. Of those, 72% reported job satisfaction either always (12%), or most of the time (60%). This indicates a relatively high degree of career satisfaction, which speaks well for APPs. However, this positive professional outlook does not reflect the whole of spiritual well-being.

Research instruments abound to measure various aspects of well-being. A recent review of 99 instruments on well-being brought attention to the vast array of measures that span a multidimensional construct for well-being (Linton, Dieppe, & Medina-Lara, 2016). This chapter identifies spiritual well-being by the two domains of life scheme and self-efficacy (Daaleman et al., 2002). A survey conducted in 2008 used these two domains to measure the spiritual well-being of PAs.

The survey audience included 777 PAs, with a response from 321 (41.3%), primarily across the Midwest (though 31 states or U.S. territories were represented). The respondents, (62.6% female, 37.4% male) completed the Spirituality Index of Well-being (Daaleman & Frey, 2004), providing a rare measure of APPs' self-report of spiritual well-being in congregate. Using 12 statements divided equally to address life scheme and self-efficacy (see Table 10.1), the PAs responded by a Likert scale from 1 to 5 (strongly agree to strongly disagree) to rate their level of agreement. Mean scores were determined, comparing PAs who worked in underserved populations with those not working with the underserved. The question of the study asked if PAs working with the underserved had a higher Spirituality Index of Well-Being (SIWB) score.

Of the PA respondents, 89 (28.6%) identified themselves as working with a state or federally designated medically underserved population (referred to as "underserved"). The mean scores for each domain, life scheme and self-efficacy, on a scale of 1 (low) to 5 (high), did not vary more than .03 between the two groups, with largely overlapping standard deviations (see Figure 10.2). When calculating the mean of both subscales for each group, the difference remained minimal and not significant (PAs-underserved 4.45 [SD = 0.48] and PAs-not underserved 4.48 [SD = 0.43]). These results suggest that in this population, the spiritual well-being of PAs was quite high, and working with the underserved did not impact the quality of well-being.

TABLE 10.1 Example Statements From the Spirituality Index of Well-Being*

Life Scheme Statements	Self-Efficacy Statements
I haven't yet found my life's purpose.	There is not much I can do to help myself.
In this world, I don't know where I fit in.	Often, there is no way I can complete what I have started.
I am far from understanding the meaning of life.	I can't begin to understand my problems.
There is a great void in my life at this time.	I am overwhelmed when I have personal difficulties or problems.

*Measured by a Likert scale from 1 (strongly agree) to 5 (strongly disagree).
Source: Daaleman and Frey (2004).

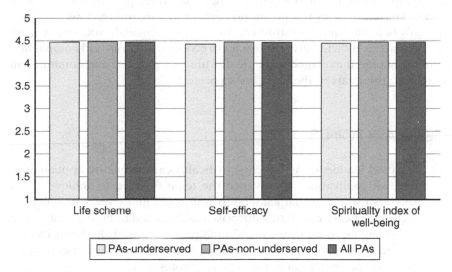

FIGURE 10.2 Results of the spirituality index of well-being from PAs (*N* = 321).
PAs, physician assistants.

DO APPS HAVE HIGH SPIRITUAL WELL-BEING?

Limitations of this study include the small sample population primarily from the Midwest states, so generalization to all PAs is not possible. The condition of voluntary participation and snowball recruitment may have skewed the results to more engaged participants. The assignment of PAs working with the "underserved" was self-reported based on formal state or federal designation, so it could not include PAs who serve in under-re-sourced populations without meeting formal designations. The study was unable to address the influence of these variables.

These data offer value in exploring how a measure can be used to measure spiritual well-being, here using the domains of life scheme and self-efficacy. Caution is required before making conclusions based on these data due to these limitations. However, the high measures found in this population raise attention to the question of spiritual well-being in different groups and locations, calling for further research.

SPIRITUAL LEADERSHIP TO DEVELOP CALLING AND MEMBERSHIP

If health care team members are struggling with a sense of purpose or belonging, spiritual leadership principles may offer guidance to the APP leader. These areas represent the powerful intrinsic motivations behind a person's behavior and therefore can be deeply personal. Addressing such essential needs individually within a team requires integrity and compassion from the leader. If managed well, greater unity of purpose and commitment to achieve the goals of the team are expected.

SUMMARY POINTS

1. Spiritual leadership is effective in health care teams by appealing to intrinsic motivations to advance the team forward to achieve goals. Leaders using spiritual leadership principles guide team members to recognize being called to a purpose (calling) and to hold a clear sense of belonging to a group (membership). Because of the integrity and compassion expected in caring for patients, spiritual leadership meets these virtues common to health care professionals.

2. Spiritual leadership skills involve casting vision, conveying hope, and practicing altruistic love. The vision is clear, idealistic, challenging, and attainable. Hope brings a sense of purpose in the midst of uncertainty (reinforcing the calling). Altruistic love instills a deep concern and appreciation for others (reinforcing membership). Exercising this combination of skills transcends the tedious obligations and distracting discouragements. The APP uses spiritual leadership skills to sincerely inspire the team to pursue extraordinary outcomes.

3. Recognizing a team's need for spiritual leadership may be difficult, and there is an abundance of different approaches to assess spiritual

well-being. A straightforward model has been exercised in health care settings based on two domains: life scheme (a person's view of the world) and self-efficacy (belief in one's own ability to perform). The APP leader gains insight by exploring the life scheme and self-efficacy of team members and creating a work environment supportive of any raised needs.

REFERENCES

Alderfer, C. P. (1969). An empirical test for a new theory of human needs. *Organizational Behavior and Human Performance, 4*, 142–175.

Bandura, A. (1997). *Self-efficacy: The exercise of control.* New York, NY: W. H. Freeman.

Daaleman, T. P., Cobb, A. K., & Frey, B. B. (2001). Spirituality and well-being: An exploratory approach to the patient perspective. *Social Science & Medicine, 53*, 119–127.

Daaleman, T. P., & Frey, B. B. (2004). The Spirituality Index of Well-Being: A new instrument for health-related quality-of-life research. *Annals of Family Medicine, 2*(5), 499–502.

Daaleman, T. P., Frey, B. B., Wallace D., & Studenski, S. A. (2002). Spirituality Index of Well-Being scale: Development and testing of a new measure. *Journal of Family Practice, 51*(11), 952.

Diener, E. (2000). Subjective well-being: The science of happiness and a proposal for a national index. *American Psychological Association, 55*, 34–43.

Donnay, D. A. C., & Borgen, F. H. (1999). The incremental validity of vocational self-efficacy: An examination of interest, self-efficacy, and occupation. *Journal of Counseling Psychology, 46*(4), 432–447.

Forrester, D. A. (2016). *Nursing's greatest leaders: A history of activism* (pp. 71–104). New York, NY: Springer Publishing.

Fry, L. W. (2003). Toward a theory of spiritual leadership. *Leadership Quarterly, 14*, 693–727.

Greenleaf, R. K. (1977). *Servant leadership* (p. 24). Mahwah, NJ: Paulist Press.

Kouzes, J., & Posner, P. (2012). *The leadership challenge: How to make extraordinary things happen in organizations.* San Francisco, CA: Jossey-Bass.

Lepnurm, R., Danielson, D., Dobson, R., & Keegan, D. (2006). Cornerstones of career satisfaction in medicine. *Canadian Psychiatric Association, 51*, 512–522.

Linton, M.-J., Dieppe, P., & Medina-Lara, A. (2016). Review of 99 self-report measures for assessing well-being in adults: Exploring dimensions of well-being and developments over time. *British Medical Journal Open, 6*, e010641. doi: 10.1136/bmjopen-2015-010641

Maslow, A. H. (1943). A theory of human motivation. In J. M. Safritz & J. S. Ott (Eds.), *Classics of organization theory* (pp. 159–173). New York, NY: Wadsworth Press. Reprinted from *Psychological Review, 50*, 370–396.

Mastain, L. (2006). The lived experience of spontaneous altruism: A phenomenological study. *Journal of Phenomenological Psychology, 37*(1), 25–52.

Maxwell, J. (2011). *The 5 levels of leadership.* New York, NY: Hachete Book Group.

Reave, L. (2005). Spiritual values and practices related to leadership effectiveness. *Leadership Quarterly, 16*, 655–687.

Ryan, R. M., & Deci, E. L. (2000). Self-determination theory and the facilitation of intrinsic motivation, social development, and well-being. *American Psychologist, 55*(1), 68–78.

Seligman, M. E. P., & Csikszentmihalyi, M. (2000). Positive psychology: An introduction. *American Psychologist, 55*(1), 5–14.

Wong, P. T. (1998). Implicit theories and the meaning of life. In P. T. Wong & P. S. Fry (Eds.), *The human quest for meaning: A handbook of psychological research and clinical applications* (pp. 111–140). Mahwah, NJ: Eribaum.

Yukl, G. (2013). *Leadership in organizations* (8th ed., p. 351). Upper Saddle River, NJ: Pearson.

11

LEADER STRATEGIES FOR TEACHING OTHERS

CRITICAL THINKING QUESTIONS

» When an advanced practice provider (APP) needs to teach the team, what instructional strategies are helpful?

» How can the APP leader help others best understand their roles in health care systems?

An oft-rewarding experience, the task of training others who newly enter the local hospital or clinic typically falls to senior APPs. The opportunity to mentor others and help shape their professional growth is a privilege; however, the new hire learns much more than clinical skills. The learner is also able to glean the APP's professional character and adopt similar values and ethics that support the principles upheld by the health care system.

APPs are encouraged to "give back" to their profession by serving as a preceptor for students just beginning their professional pursuits. While this is admirable and the professional educators are thankful, the rewards are even greater when the APP is able to teach members of the team. The exclusive, local value gained when APPs effectively guide an individual forward professionally within their health care team promises a productive relational structure, building dependable communication ties.

Without need for declaration, APP leaders should assume this role of a *teacher* to their team members. The ability to lead effectively depends on the skills of the APP to help the team understand systems, apply strategies, and critically reason to reach team goals and deliver high-quality patient care. APP leaders must facilitate team members in learning these expectations to advance forward.

CASE STUDY 1

Anya is a 30-year-old nurse practitioner (NP) employed full time by a suburban pediatric practice with five physicians and three other APPs. She has been with the practice for 7 years, first as a registered nurse (RN) and now as an NP the past 3 years. She is meeting Derek, a newly hired PA, and he will accompany her for the next 3 days to become oriented to the flow of patient care delivery, electronic medical records, and the scope of the practice.

Derek is in his mid-40s, recently retired from 27 years in the U.S. Air Force. He was educated as a physician assistant (PA) in the military and has 15 years of clinical practice, including three tours in the Middle East, and most recently 2 years at a West Coast base providing family medical care for soldiers and their families.

Anya met Derek earlier when he interviewed for the position. His clinical experience included high levels of patient responsibility with impressive stories of mass trauma and complicated health conditions. A likable man, his more recent years in family medicine offered sufficient pediatric experience that the practice agreed to hire him with an understanding that he would have a learning curve in acclimating to their pediatric practice.

Anya is apprehensive over Derek's broad clinical experience compared to her own, but also appreciates the confidence the practice has placed in her to help Derek get off to a solid start. She is exploring how she should best help Derek adjust to pediatric care.

There is an assumption that a new adult employee best learns a new role by coming alongside an experienced coworker who models desired behaviors and skills. That method of learning works well in many technical and industrial functions. The APP must recognize that much more is required in orienting a new coworker beyond just tasks and skills.

In Case Study 1, Anya recognizes she needs to help Derek understand the practice of pediatrics as distinct from family medicine or other specialties. She also understands the scope of care provided by the pediatric office in this local community, the expectations that patients and families have for the providers, and the expectations the providers communicate to their patient population. Management patterns for acute care needs, well-child checks, and chronic care needs of their patients are examples of the many aspects of care Anya must share with Derek as a part of his orientation.

Anya is largely responsible for Derek's success in his first days of employment. An orderly approach to assume this teacher role will bring a more rewarding outcome for both Anya and Derek.

CONDITIONS OF LEARNING IN PRACTICE

Robert M. Gagné (1916–2002) was an American educational psychologist who established several models of learning processes that continue to have application with adult learners today. First published in 1965, his text, *Conditions of Learning* (1977), remains a classic volume of education theory with application. Gagné started with an assumption that there are different types of learning so that instruction needs to be different to support various learning styles. Three steps of instruction framed his approach to learning:

1. Break up the content of instruction into components.

2. Gain mastery of each component.

3. Sequence the components to lead to the goal of learning.

Applying these steps, Anya would benefit from making a list of general concepts and tasks that Derek will need to learn and create a logical, realistic order for his learning. Gagné offers models for learning to help guide Anya.

Categories of Learning

Five categories of learning define different types of information and skills (Gagné originally called these "varieties of learning," 1977). Each category holds unique methods for learning and requires different strategies of instruction (see Table 11.1).

» **Verbal information:** This employs rote memorization, such as Derek needing to learn pediatric immunization schedules.

» **Intellectual skills:** This represents information that requires some degree of thinking and reasoning, such as a pediatric clinic's management of recurrent otitis media. A group pediatric practice may follow a uniform system of antibiotic usage, and Anya can explain generally adopted protocols or treatment principles recommended by this local office.

» **Cognitive strategies:** This presents information that is more complex, requiring clinical reasoning skills. Examples in Anya's practice setting may be the strategy of evaluating pediatric abdominal pain, use of lab and imaging studies, consulting with pediatricians, and consideration of hospitalization and referrals.

» **Motor skills:** This category involves cognitive thinking and doing. Anya identifies wart treatment at her clinic as a common motor skill using in-office cryotherapy by the providers when indicated.

» **Attitudes:** Derek will need to learn how to approach certain common, challenging situations. Anya will need to convey to Derek the pediatric practice's philosophy in dealing with families who are insistent on receiving antibiotics without appropriate indications. Another example is discussing with Derek the approach to suspected child abuse to help him be familiar with the local resources and approach.

In some situations, the new APP may enter a situation and find that there are not sufficient resources or people assigned to help guide the needed learning. The APP may need to request this support and offer to develop a process for learning for a more complete and efficient orientation (see Exercise 11.1 later in this chapter).

TABLE 11.1 Gagné's Categories of Learning for Clinicians*

Category*	Content to Learn	Clinical Content Example	Learning Strategy
Verbal information	Terms and lists	Names, formulary, E&M codes	Use of visual cues, mnemonics
Intellectual skills	Problem-solving concrete concepts	EMR use, lab orders, scheduling system	Build on prior learning, repetition
Cognitive strategy	Requires critical thinking and clinical reasoning	Triaging, referral, consultations	Return-demonstration with varying scenarios
Attitude	A choice of action toward a situation	Managing angry patients, telling bad news	Simulation or role-play with feedback
Motor skills	Behavioral physical skills	Surgical instrumentation skills, sterile technique	Visual demonstration, practice with immediate feedback

E&M, evaluation and management; EMR, electronic medical record.
*Categories are from Gagné et al. (2004).

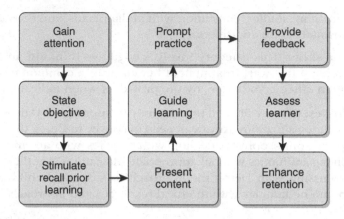

FIGURE 11.1 Nine events of instruction (Gagné).
Source: From GAGNE. The Conditions of Learning, 3E. © 1977 South-Western, a part of Cengage, Inc. Reproduced by permission. www.cengage.com/permissions.

Events of Instruction

Gagné presented nine Events of Instruction as a stepwise process of planned instruction (Gagné, Wager, Golas, & Keller, 2004). While on-the-job training does not require extensive, planned instruction, Gagné's principles offer a straightforward framework for effective learning in the clinical environment (as well as in the classroom). The APP with responsibility to teach team members will benefit from efficiently using an orderly approach to facilitate clinical learning such as presented here (see Figure 11.1). In addition to Gagné's nine steps, two additional steps (numbered 10 and 11 in the following list) may have particular value in bedside teaching (Al-Eraky, 2012).

1. **Gain attention:** Use a question or interesting statistic to alert the learner to something new.

2. **State objective:** Discuss expectations of what is to be learned and what level of mastery is anticipated.

3. **Stimulate recall of prior learning:** Use a recent patient or other background knowledge to begin a framework on which the learner can build.

4. **Present content:** Demonstrate the skill or disclose the new content.

5. **Guide learning:** Have the learner rehearse the steps of the skill or suggest helpful cues that broaden understanding.

6. **Prompt practice:** With or without direct guidance, give time for the learner to study content or practice the skill now or later.

7. **Provide feedback:** Respond to questions and offer informative feedback.

8. **Assess learner:** By observation or a more formal means, evaluate the learner's achievement of the goals of learning. This may require more feedback with repeated assessment to gain mastery.

9. **Enhance retention and transfer:** Reiterate the value of what is learned and explore other situations that utilize this knowledge or skill.

10. **Suggest resources:** Recommend additional readings, media resources, or links to deepen learning.

11. **Discussion:** While discussion occurs throughout all the steps, a focused time of interactive discussion between the teacher and learner augments the learning experience for both parties.

Each of the 11 steps holds value, but individual steps may not apply, or a single action may meet multiple steps. Tailoring this system to the unique learning environment fosters an efficient and orderly process of instruction.

EXERCISE 11.1 QUESTIONS FOR THE APP

For students who have their professional positions yet ahead, or APPs who are considering a change of employment, the following exercise may be helpful in exploring a new APP role.

1. *Select the employment specialty or setting desired.*

2. *Using Gagné's categories of learning, identify what content in the potential employment would be important to understand for a new APP. Use the examples given in this chapter related to Case Study 1 (the content Anya has determined is needed for Derek to begin the pediatric practice) as a guide.*

3. *If possible, contact an APP from that specialty or setting and interview him or her using the following questions as a model for each category of learning:*

   a. *Verbal information: What knowledge do you use in your specific practice that has to be memorized? Are there commonly used lists or reference points?*

   b. *Intellectual skills: What is the general pattern of your day/ week? How are schedules organized? What diagnostic or*

> *treatment technology such as lab and imaging are available for immediate use versus referral?*
>
> c. *Cognitive strategies: Do you have any stories that describe how a more complex patient is directed through a referral or consultation?*
>
> d. *Attitude: How do you handle patients who are noncompliant or have difficult attitudes?*
>
> e. *Motor skills: If I were new to this specialty or setting, what skills would I need to master to be fully acclimated to this position?*

SOCIAL COGNITIVE THEORY

A second significant issue raised in Case Study 1 is Anya's insecurity about orienting a PA who has twice the years of experience as her own. Derek's military experience as a PA far exceeded her own experience according to the stories he told of managing patients with multiple trauma and highly complex health care needs. Anya's only health care experience has been at this same pediatric clinic, first as a nurse and then as an NP. While she has seen a wide variety of pediatric conditions, she has not dealt with the types of clinical challenges Derek has had over his military service. She wonders if she will be intimidated in trying to teach Derek about pediatric clinical practice and questions if he should rather be teaching her.

Anya's perspective implies that she views learning occurring when the teacher dispenses knowledge and the student absorbs it. This more simplistic view of learning is in parallel with some older, outdated theories of learning that suggested an input–output process of education that applied to early days of computer programming (e.g., the information-processing theory). Progressive education theories represent different and more effective processes of learning, useful in conceptualizing the role of the leader in adult learning environments.

Social Cognitive Theory (SCT), authored by Albert Bandura (1989), builds on the premise that learning occurs by observing others. He argued that an individual does not learn autonomously, nor is learning a mechanical process. SCT finds that learning occurs when an individual is engaged in a reciprocal influence with at least one and likely a combination of the environment, the behaviors of others, and the cognition skills of others.

1. **The environment:** An invigorating environment tailored to the learner provides for effective learning. A modern health care facility offers an environment that stimulates greater learning by the surrounding professional culture supporting health care delivery. A supportive

environment for learning includes consideration of the size of the room, furniture to sit in, use of technology (e.g., access to useful media), color schemes, and ambient temperature. It may be conducive to learning to step away from a highly visual, active environment and learn in a more subdued location, such as a coffee shop or other quieter locale.

2. **Behavior:** Observing the behaviors of others during instruction is integral to learning according to SCT. Social experiences and interactions are powerful influences on learning. Among clinicians, the mannerisms and behaviors observed between each other communicates important nonverbal concepts of knowledge applications, identity, and culture. Sharing past health care experiences or previously learned cues on disease management stimulates a more dynamic atmosphere that engages those involved and enhances learning.

3. **Cognition:** Observing how someone else is learning is a strong influence on learning. If the instructor provides ideas for how to learn a concept, or the learner is able to compare strategies for learning a skill with someone else (e.g., asking questions, organizing information, and voicing self-reflection with others), everyone benefits.

Self-Efficacy and SCT

Key to Anya's success in orienting Derek is her level of self-efficacy (discussed in Chapter 10 as one of the two domains measured in spiritual well-being). Self-efficacy is an individual's belief in the capacity to organize and perform tasks necessary to achieve a goal (Bandura, 1997). Anya needs high self-efficacy to orient Derek, just as Derek needs self-efficacy to learn his new role. This is a key component of SCT as the social interaction between the teacher and other learners is necessary to grow self-efficacy.

Enhanced self-efficacy decreases anxiety and tension while increasing a positive mood. This is a recognized concept in patient care and plays a significant role as a mediator between knowledge and action toward healthy behaviors (Bandura, 2004). For example, patients who lose weight or stop smoking likely achieved these goals because of high self-efficacy.

By her awareness of self-efficacy, Anya should gain confidence in her ability to orient Derek and enjoy the benefit of engaging his past experience in the learning environment. Understanding that she will learn from Derek based on his prior experience, and Derek will learn from Anya about the local pediatric practice, SCT establishes a framework for this effective learning relationship.

The strength of SCT in establishing a model for effective learning is dependent on four actions that support self-efficacy (see Table 11.2). The

TABLE 11.2 Self-Efficacy Exercises

Teacher Action	Method	Expected Learner Response
Mastery experiences	Rehearsal and practice	"I did it."
Vicarious experiences	Success stories of others	"If they can do it, so can I."
Verbal persuasion	Messages of encouragement	"She believes I can do it."
Feedback on progress	Correction and support	"I can do it correctly."

APP should use a combination of these actions when facilitating a team member's learning and development:

» **Provide experiences for mastery:** Allow the learner to practice learning and show achievement.

» **Provide vicarious experiences:** Tell stories of how others have had success in learning as a model of desired expectations.

» **Encourage success:** Give messages of encouragement to keep the learner advancing forward.

» **Provide feedback:** Positive feedback and correction are needed and should be provided often and, if possible, immediately.

Leaders are positioned to help their team members reach higher levels of self-efficacy, and the four aforementioned actions may help.

In Case Study 1, Anya's own self-efficacy as a leader is also in need of support. The demands of leadership bring moments when self-doubt occurs regarding the leader's own abilities. While expected to support the self-efficacy of their team members, the leader faces difficult situations creating personal feelings of inadequacy. The aforementioned four actions still apply, accomplished by self-reflection. The leader can rehearse a role (mastery experiences), recall past experiences of success (vicarious experiences), give reassuring self-talks (encourage success), and self-assess with advice (provide feedback).

If a trusted mentor is available, seeking counsel is appropriate when self-doubts arise. However, the self-aware leader may find that putting these principles into mental practice oneself will bolster the leadership required.

CONCEPTUALIZING HEALTH CARE SYSTEMS

All members of today's health care team must be knowledgeable about health care systems. Because of the rapidity of change as health care reform continues in the mix of complex systems, the team must be nimble to adjust to challenges, revisions, and enhancements. New members to the health care team will help the team be effective if they are highly functioning in direct patient care while staying responsive to the broad scope of systems management, including reimbursement, quality control, patient and employee safety, and population health outcomes.

These broader issues of health care systems are neglected when the focus is solely on how to treat an individual patient. With the priority of patient care sustained, the APP must appreciate internal and external influences on the local health care system. The APP in leadership is responsible to ensure that the health care team is fully informed.

One method the leader can use to help the team comprehend the broader scope of health care delivery is to guide the consideration of local system issues and challenges through Bolman and Deal's Leadership Frameworks (2013). Four perspectives (frames) for understanding organizations cover different angles by which issues can affect a system. The frames serve as lenses that help focus on pertinent concerns, avoiding an otherwise blurred understanding that may seem overwhelming.

CASE STUDY 2

Seth is an APP leading a hospitalist team of eight professionals providing interprofessional care. He has just learned that one of their most valuable members, Claire, has resigned her role to relocate with her partner to another state. She has met with all team members to express her appreciation for their support and great working relationships. Seth has since learned that the team is discouraged as there is no clear candidate readily available to fill Claire's role. The team dynamics are going to change and the uncertainty is causing significant stress. Seth believes there is now a risk of other team departures over this discontent that he must prevent. He calls a meeting to help the team process Claire's absence and explore future prospects.

Seth chooses to use the Leadership Framework to guide the team through the consequences expected with Claire's departure. The frames cover four perspectives: structural, human resource, political, and symbolic.

» **Structural:** The structural aspects of the team include assigned roles, strategy and goals, and the degree of order and control exercised. When goals are clear, roles are covered and efforts are orderly and systematic, the structural frame is intact. Uncertainly, ambiguity and conflict create weaknesses in the structural frame.

» **Human resource:** This frame emphasizes the support and empowerment of people on the team. The needs, feelings, talents, and limitations of the team members are recognized and addressed. The human resource frame depends on a team that feels good about what they are doing. Low morale and interpersonal conflict weaken this frame.

» **Political:** Competing power bases and interest groups constitute this frame, dependent on effective coalition building, negotiating, and compromise. If a dominant (internal or external) force is in conflict with the team's values, the political frame is unstable.

» **Symbolic:** The vision and inspiration of the team holds the symbolic frame intact. Evidence of traditions, celebrations, and other rituals supports this frame. When the team goals or directions are unclear, this frame may suffer.

Application of the leadership framework helps the team explore an issue and consider ramifications and potential consequences to address while also identifying dependable strengths. A study of the use of this framework when facing critical incidents found that structural frames were used most often and symbolic frames the least (Bolman & Deal, 1991). The authors of the framework recommend that all four frameworks be functional to comprehensively understand and respond to the influence of issues.

CASE STUDY 2 (CONTINUED)

Seth assembled his team and presented the four leadership frameworks. In light of Claire's departure, he asked the team to discuss strengths and weaknesses according to each frame. Their results were as follows:

- *Structural: With Claire leaving, one person cannot currently assume her role so several members will need to have roles reassigned to cover her responsibilities.*

- *Human resource: Replacing Claire is a priority, but the team agrees that it is critical to take the time necessary to find a person who has a similar team-player attitude and strong clinical skills. The team agreed that experience was not as critical a factor as character; the team would be committed to training the right person.*

- *Political: The team feared the administration would maintain high expectations for their productivity in Claire's absence, requiring other members to take extra shifts.*

- *Symbolic: The team felt they could sustain this loss as long as they remain unified in purpose and a new person was found reasonably soon to fill the opening. They agreed to hold a farewell party for Claire and be sure she was recognized for her many contributions to the team.*

From this meeting, Seth gained direction for his leadership. He told the team that based on this helpful analysis he would focus on two of the four frames: structure (making temporary reassignments and initiating a candidate search for Claire's replacement) and political (speaking with administration to be sure reasonable expectations were granted to the team while they were down a team member). Seth remarked to the team that he would depend on the strengths of the human resource and symbolic frames (the team agreed to hold steady until they find the right replacement). He suggested they meet as a team again in a week to review the status of these four frames.

Giving value to all four frames gives the team a comprehensive perspective on issues that arise. Using this process to help the team understand the broader implications across the health care system will lead to a more informed and thoughtful direction.

LEADER AS TEACHER

While often more implied than said, the leader of a health care team is often fulfilling the role of a teacher. This role can be delegated if others with teaching skills are available, but the education of the team to accomplish its goals still falls to the APP leader. With an understanding of SCT, the tools of Gagné's events of instruction, the support of self-efficacy, and the viewpoint of Bolman and Deal's Leadership Frameworks, the APP leader has helpful resources to support the teaching role.

SUMMARY POINTS

1. APPs have opportunities to orient new staff, provide training in procedures, and introduce updated processes to the health care team. Assuming this role of "teacher" is encouraged, and a number of

instructional strategies are available to maximize learning. For adult learners, recognizing that learning is a social construct involving a person interacting with others and the environment guides the APP's approach to teaching. This differs from the archaic model of a distinct separation between teacher and student. Today's "student" benefits from reciprocal interactions, such as the APP sharing information to be learned, discussing the topic for feedback, exchanging strategies, and exploring questions. The social cognitive theory of learning provides an opportunity to build up the self-efficacy of the learner (a personal belief in one's ability to perform). When there is a significant amount of content to learn or an important skill to master, the APP will find it helpful to organize the learning process. Gagné's Events of Instruction or similar framework provides structure to make the most of the learning opportunity.

2. The complexities and challenges in today's health care systems require the team to be knowledgeable and adept in working within the local system. The APP must be able to provide excellent patient care and support the multifaceted work of the health care team so that the outcomes meet community health goals, are cost-effective, support access to care, and maintain patient satisfaction. The APP leader serves the team by helping members understand and value their contribution to the larger health care system. Teaching about the complexities of health care delivery includes focused applications about the role the health care team from different perspectives. Bolman and Deal's Leadership Frameworks offer four viewpoints (structural, human resource, political, and symbolic) that the APP leader can use to guide the team in appreciating the breadth of health care the system needs and the team's role.

REFERENCES

Al-Eraky, M. M. (2012). Robert Gagné's nine events of instruction, revisited. *Academic Medicine, 87*(5), 677.

Bandura, A. (1989). Social cognitive theory. In R. Vasta, (Ed.), *Annals of child development: Six theories of child development* (Vol. 6, pp. 1–60). Greenwich, CT: JAI Press.

Bandura, A. (1997). *Self-efficacy: The exercise of control.* New York, NY: W. H. Freeman.

Bandura, A. (2004). Health promotion by social cognitive means. *Health Education & Behavior, 31*(2), 143–164.

Bolman, L. G., & Deal, T. E. (1991). Leadership and management effectiveness: A multi-frame, multi-sector analysis. *Human Resource Management, 30*(4), 509–534.

Bolman, L. G., & Deal, T. E. (2013). *Reframing organizations: Artistry, choice & leadership* (5th ed.). San Franciso, CA: Jossey-Bass.

Gagné, R. M. (1977). *The conditions of learning* (3rd ed.). Stamford, CT: Thomson.

Gagné, R. M., Wager, W. W., Golas, K., & Keller, J. M. (2004). *Principles of instructional design* (5th ed.). Belmont, CA: Wadsworth.

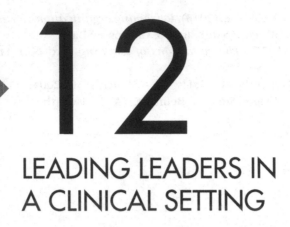

12

LEADING LEADERS IN A CLINICAL SETTING

CRITICAL THINKING QUESTIONS

» **What leadership skills can advanced practice providers (APPs) use to guide a physician or other leader to consider alternative courses of action?**

» **When steering a health care team, what can the APP leader do to help the team be nimble and adaptable?**

» **How does an APP lead a more complex team whose members are all leaders of their own teams?**

APPs function with a high level of responsibility in patient care that 50 years ago resided only in the hands of a physician. In the early days of the APP professions, physicians delegated patient care duties to nurse practitioners (NPs) and physician assistants (PAs). As physicians entrusted greater responsibility to APPs, the "team" approach developed and expanded in each profession, with a gradual shift from a prevailing physician leader to today's collaborative care teams.

HELPING OTHER LEADERS

NPs and PAs followed distinct courses to reach this point in their respective professional evolutions, but the endpoint is comparable. APPs now provide direct patient care to a substantial portion of the U.S. population

(Essary, Green, & Gans, 2016; Morgan, Everett, & Hing, 2015). Replacing the autocratic physician role of the past are different and varied leader models coordinated within interdisciplinary teams, resulting in shared leadership.

For example, the solo APP in an isolated rural setting is able to influence surrounding physicians, community leaders, public health officials, and others. The APP on a subspecialty surgical team is able to influence surgeons, other members across the team, hospital administrators, and health care coordinators. APPs who are skilled in contributing to the leadership of other leaders broaden the influence of their role and perspective for more effective, high-quality health care delivery with improved patient outcomes.

Case Study 1 offers an example of patient care at a local level from an APP who avoided this leadership role, placing patient safety at risk.

CASE STUDY 1

[This is recounted as a true story by a physician assistant.]

I was in my first days of a new job and met one of the family practice physicians early in the morning to accompany him on morning rounds. A beloved community physician, he was congenial and introduced me to each patient as a new partner on the team. I was privileged to work with him and had long admired his reputation. Just before we entered a new mom's room, he briefed me that she had delivered the morning before and would be dismissed today. In the room, we learned from the nurse rounding with us that the mom had an indwelling urinary catheter placed last night because she could not void. The nurse reported that the patient this morning was otherwise doing well. He frowned his disapproval about the decision to place the catheter. We entered the room and after introductions said empathetically to the patient, "You don't need that catheter now. We'll remove it so you can go home." The nurse left to go get what was needed as he continued a brief physical examination.

Finishing his examination of her abdomen, the doctor softly asked his patient, "It's uncomfortable, isn't it?" The mom nodded and he responded, "Let's just get it out." He proceeded to pull on the end of the urinary catheter to remove it.

I saw the catheter stretch but it held tightly inside the woman's bladder.

Standing across the room, I immediately recognized that the bladder of the catheter wasn't deflated. The doctor pulled again and looked quizzically at me when again he found resistance. He paused and firmly said, "It should really come out." Then he gave a strong pull, bringing the catheter fully out, with the patient yelping discomfort. Only then was it clear to him that the balloon on the catheter now dangling from his hand was still fully inflated.

I can be hard on the doctor; he should have known the catheter balloon needed to be deflated. But, I'm wondering why I didn't say anything. I guess I was intimidated a bit by it being my first days on the job. I suppose I thought he knew what he was doing, but I knew what the problem was. Why didn't I speak up?

In 1999, the Institute of Medicine (IOM) released *To Err Is Human: Building a Safer Health System.* This stirred a national awareness of medical errors contributing to significant patient morbidity and mortality. The IOM report guided health care leaders to avoid being consumed by concerns of incompetency, poor work ethic, or medical errors, as, by and large, these were not the causes of the vast majority of poor patient outcomes. The solution is not found in pointing fingers or overly cautioning the team to "be more careful."

Instead, the IOM called for a new culture of patient and employee safety that remains the challenge today. A culture of safety includes developing an environment that explores latent factors that contribute to errors such as those noted in Case Study 1. In that situation, factors include provider fatigue, lack of procedural process, and an overdependence on one's memory or vigilance. In addition, the APP in that Case Study raises the factor of a missed opportunity to intervene. This latter factor, which could have prevented the medical error if only the APP would have spoken up, occurred because of insecurities in the APP and a health care team dynamic that did not foster having the APP intervene.

Since the IOM report, many programs have been created and implemented throughout U.S. institutions to develop the culture of safety. Evidence documents the success of teamwork in improving the quality, safety, and cost-effectiveness of health care delivery (e.g., Salas et al., 2009).

One of these patient safety programs, TeamSTEPPS®, sponsored by the Agency for Healthcare Research and Quality (AHRQ), supports the team development of four skills: communication, leadership, situation monitoring, and mutual support. To successfully learn these skills, the team must first work together effectively in advancing a culture of safety (based on mutual trust and a shared mental model). Once these characteristics of the team are established, these four skills become the focus of TeamSTEPPS (see Table 12.1).

TABLE 12.1 Elements of TeamSTEPPS 2.0 Curriculum

Team Structure Components	Communication Skills	Leadership Skills	Situation Monitoring	Mutual Support
Patient	Critical information communication techniques:	Leader responsibilities	Shared mental model	Protect from overload
Core team	• Key components	Team events to implement plan:	Status of patient	Ask for and offer assistance
Coordinating team	• Directing communication	• Sharing the plan	Team members	Performance feedback
Ancillary and support services	Closed-loop communication	• Monitoring/ modifying the plan	Environment	Advocacy for patient
Administration	Patient handoff communication	• Reviewing the team's work	Progress	Manage conflict

Source: Adapted from *TeamSTEPPS 2.0* (2015).

» **Communication:** Using a structured process that includes a shared mental model, information is clearly and accurately exchanged.

» **Leadership:** The leadership of the team assures the availability of resources; all members understand team actions and any changes are shared across the team.

» **Situation monitoring:** The team has a developed process for scanning and assessing all elements of the workplace to support effective team function.

» **Mutual support:** Needs of team members are anticipated and supported, balancing responsibilities and workloads.

The TeamSTEPPS skill of communication offers guidance to establish a developed culture of safety on a team (Sheppard, Williams, & Klein, 2013). This skill includes the team learning to exercise clear communication. For example, when questions are asked, clear responses are given (e.g., Leader: *Airway status?* – Team member: *Airway clear.*). When orders are given, they are checked in a closed-loop dialog (e.g., Leader: *Give 5 mg morphine IV.* – Team member: *5 mg morphine.* – Leader: *That's correct.*). TeamSTEPPS also institutes clear communication processes for patient handoffs (a significant factor in medical errors) and communication of critical information.

The skill of mutual support as guided by TeamSTEPPS helps reduce the risk of errors. The training content describes the team member's role as an advocate for the patient, establishing a communication process for intervening when a team member differs in opinion or action from the leader. The team is taught a culture of asserting corrective action with respect, empowering all team members to stop the action if there is a safety issue. Among other processes, the TeamSTEPPS curriculum teaches the team to recognize and say progressively assertive statements in the face of potential patient harm, such as:

» I am concerned!

» I am uncomfortable!

» This is a safety issue!

The TeamSTEPPS curriculum or similar programs are useful to help leaders and team members together create an environment that protects patients and the health care team.

LEADING LEADERS OF HEALTH CARE TEAMS

This text has explored a variety of leadership strategies to support APPs in contributing leadership skills in a variety of health care systems. Because of the development of more and more complex systems, the associated teams within these systems are structured within necessarily convoluted pathways. Within these health care grids, individuals hold leadership roles overseeing leaders of other teams. APPs are assuming these roles, leading leaders.

Defining a Team

A "team" has many different forms without consistency. The physician who has employed a PA to deliver patient care but then rarely interacts with the PA is not a model of a functional team. At its core, a team should be at least two individuals who share a common purpose by using their complementary skills with mutual accountability (Morrison, Goldfarb, & Lanken, 2010). As the team expands with more individuals and talents, the organization of the team will vary, with roles of leadership distributed and shared. When weaknesses occur within the team, other team members step up so that the sum of the team's abilities becomes greater than the parts. As APPs assume leadership roles, it is common to find them working with many leaders from other teams as well as their own.

Team Development

Tuckman and Jensen (1977) presented five stages of team development that remain popularly recognized by the terms: forming, storming, norming, performing, and adjourning (see Table 12.2). An early team usually finds members on their best behavior (forming stage), but as the group begins to work together, frustrations surface (storming) as personalities and perceived roles are in conflict. As the team learns to develop consensus (norming), they understand each member's contributions and work well together (performing). Recognizing that a team has an endpoint, the final stage indicates a termination of the original team as it grows with membership changes and responsibilities (adjourning).

Each stage is associated with a leadership strategy, starting with the leader coordinating the forming stage, coaching the storming stage, empowering the norming and performing stages, and supporting the adjourning stage (Manges, Scott-Cawiezell, & Ward, 2017). APP leaders who recognize these stages, both in their own teams and when working with other teams, will be better able to direct teams in working together.

Team Competencies

Successful teams reflect functional competencies that build on various strengths of team members. When the team comprises a group of leaders,

TABLE 12.2 Stages of Team Development

Developmental Stage*	Qualities	Leadership Strategy**
Forming	Exploring roles, leader dependent	Coordinating
Storming	Defining roles creates friction, raises anxieties	Coaching
Norming	Cohesive roles bring collective strengths	Empowering
Performing	Functioning roles achieve goals	Empowering
Adjourning	Roles expand, original team unrecognizable	Supporting

*Adapted from Tuckman and Jensen (1977).
**Adapted from Manges et al. (2017).

it is imperative that the members give attention to the competencies to clarify roles and avoid leader conflict. Three categories of competencies include knowledge, skills, and attitudes, represented in the team as a whole (Morrison et al., 2010).

> » **Knowledge competencies:** The team understands its mission and tasks, and general access to resources. The team recognizes each member's characteristics with distribution of roles fitting personalities and demands.

> » **Skills competencies:** The team holds mutual accountability that members are contributing to the work, responding to individual needs with coaching and feedback, managing challenges and conflict.

> » **Attitude competencies:** The team has a shared vision with high self-efficacy and trust as a group. The team recognizes they are better as a collective than as individuals and work to resolve conflict.

LEADERSHIP RESEARCH CHALLENGES

Evidence from leadership research is difficult to secure to guide leaders in managing a complex team or multiple teams. Leadership studies explore theories within a small group or more likely in a dyadic relationship of leader and follower. It is well recognized among leadership researchers that their methods are often based on questionable assumptions (Yukl, 2013) and unique environments that limit the portability of results.

Observations of leadership behaviors often come from surveys or focus group interviews that retrospectively rate leader effectiveness. These results have limited validity and reliability as the participants carry bias that often inflates favor or disfavor toward the leader. Scholars support more qualitative research methods to provide a greater depth of study into the characteristics of applied leadership. However, standards of evaluation are not explicit in qualitative studies, allowing considerable freedom in the researchers' interpretation of findings. Studies that are intensive and longitudinal with data collection from at least two different perspectives (interviews, observations, open-ended surveys, performance records) strengthen the credibility of the research.

In today's elaborate and sophisticated health care systems, the APP leader should review leadership models through a critical lens that considers the unique elements of his or her own leadership style, situation, team, and resources.

ACHIEVING ORGANIZATIONAL HEALTH

Lencioni (2012) coined the term "organizational health" for a team that fits together well in its operations and strategies. He distinguishes the *healthy* organization from the *smart* organization. Much attention is given to a team's strategy, finances, technology, and, in the business sector, marketing. A smart team would support each of these. However, the characteristics expected in a healthy team are high productivity, low turnover, high morale, and minimal politics and confusion. These latter attributes should be the focus of the APP leader. If those are in place, the team will likely find success at being healthy.

CASE STUDY 2

Mona is an APP who has worked at a university-based tertiary care center in an endocrinology specialty for 12 years. Her group includes eight physicians and six other APPs. She manages the schedule for all providers and by default of seniority is the APP to whom the doctors and department administrators come when discussing APP utilization in the clinic and hospital, patient traffic and satisfaction, and other human or technical resources that involve APPs.

With a history of performing well in her position, seen as approachable and wise, Mona holds the respect of many across the institution. This brings Mona to today's meeting with her department administrator, the physician department head, and the chief medical officer (CMO) of the institution. They are recommending that Mona be appointed to a new position as chief APP officer (or CAP) for the institution. The CMO has previously been responding to many inquiries for increased utilization of APPs across most departments, advancing hospitalist teams in units that do not yet have them, and staffing new outlying clinics associated with the university. He mentions that the institution is aware that it is not appropriately billing for APP services in many departments (she and other APPs have known this for some time) and that this would need focused attention. The CMO has attended national conferences that have featured the topic of APP administration and recognizes that for an institution of this size, it is behind others in this progression of administrative leadership.

The CMO is committed to training Mona, sending her to institutions that have already established APP central offices and to conferences for additional education. The enormity of the task would require that she step away from her clinical practice for at least 1 year, and would begin meeting with the other department heads to learn the breadth and scope of APP utilization and needs. She would also meet directly with all APPs and determine how best to organize her office to be responsive to their inquiries and needs.

Mona's department administrator shares that while the department would sorely miss her, he believes she is the right fit for this role based on how she has managed the APPs around her. The physician department head agrees, and states that after a year, the CMO and he would meet with Mona to discuss possible arrangements for her to return part-time to continue patient care in the department, should she wish to continue her clinical practice. The CMO shares that he believes establishing the APP office is a 2-year project, but after the first year, he would consider the distribution of responsibilities and progress made, so that, if Mona missed clinical practice, they would try to support her part-time return.

The CMO asks that if salary and employment arrangements were satisfactory, would she consider this opportunity.

The APP Leader for a Healthy Team

Facilitating effective teams that readily adapt to changes in the health care system is the goal of the APP leader. The leadership skills for a larger team or multiple teams include problem solving and material resource management, but the majority of the leader's time focuses on managing personnel. To manage personnel well, the leader establishes an effective team structure and role placement, followed by coaching the members and reinforcing a compelling vision (Burke et al., 2006).

Leadership styles that are most effective for these personnel needs include person-focused behaviors compared to task-focused behaviors. This is supported by leadership behaviors that empower the team (e.g., transformational, servant, and adaptive leadership styles), rather than transactional leadership styles. In Case Study 2, Mona needs to explore her own leadership style, recognize her own skills, and determine if she is ready to devote more attention to exercising her leadership in the development of this APP office.

Healthy Meetings

The bane of leadership is directing and attending a number of various meetings. While no activity receives more criticism, there is also no better method of sustaining the health of the team. As taking a temperature assesses a patient's vital signs, observing a meeting led by an APP assesses the vitality of the team.

The APP leader is advised to be intentional in planning meetings under his or her control, and consider four types of meetings common to healthy organizations: administrative, tactical, strategic, and developmental meetings (Lencioni, 2012).

» **Administrative meetings:** These are daily visits of 5 to 10 minutes, as long as the team can be assembled conveniently at one location or by technology. Avoid strict agendas: the purpose is to keep the team talking. Minor issues can be quickly resolved before they fester, and information is collected on larger, looming issues for later discussion.

» **Tactical meetings:** This is the routine weekly meeting (45–90 minutes) of the team. Lencioni suggests a real-time agenda where the meeting opens with team members each offering quick item topics that need discussion. Within 5 to 10 minutes, a list of topics is developed and the team can together address the topics by priority. Compelling topics that require more time for a thoughtful discussion are postponed for presentation at the next strategic meeting (see next meeting type).

» **Strategic meetings:** These occur as needed, typically requiring 2 to 4 hours to address critical topics that have a long-term effect on the health care system. These meetings may require some prior data gathering so that solutions can be thoughtfully addressed after debate. The leader finds these meetings often most rewarding; however, they are at risk of being neglected due to busy schedules. Assuring that strategic topics are viewed as critical and discussion brings specific actions can make these the most valuable and anticipated meetings of the team.

» **Developmental meetings:** Getting the team offsite on a quarterly basis for a day (or two) will meet administrative resistance as expensive due to the loss of productivity or revenue from those attending and requiring rented space, meals, travel, and other costs. The leader must be able to argue that the benefits outweigh these costs, such as the anticipated gains of team cohesiveness, operational responses to significant threats, revisions of long-term strategies, and necessary planning for cost-saving technologies or processes. Meetings facilitated by a trusted outside consultant allow the team leader to participate equally alongside the team.

Maximizing the work of the team by leading productive meetings is the leader's frequent responsibility. The APP leader who facilitates meetings that members find useful and that bring results will advance the team to reach its goals.

LEADING TEAMS IN COMPLEX SYSTEMS

The future of health care is expected to only become more complex. Interwoven challenges of the growing size of populations needing care, continual and welcome advancements to treat conditions, unpredictable new pathogens and other insults to health, and avenues for improved preventive care will continue to bring greater demands on currently strained health care systems.

A model for leadership among complex military teams based in the convoluted environment of the Iraq war of 2004 was developed, described by General Stanley McChrystal, Collins, Silverman, and Fussell (2015). McChrystal is a former commander of the U.S. and International Security Assistance Forces in Afghanistan and the former commander of the Joint Special Operations Command.

While military models of leadership are often hierarchical and highly structured, McChrystal found that with the chaos of the environment and the unorthodox actions of enemy forces, the traditional hierarchy had to change. While his team utilized the latest and best technology and orchestrated honed tactics of war, it was ineffective in battling this enemy. The unpredictability of the environment was incompatible with a leadership model built from estimated forecasts and strategic planning.

McChrystal generated two key principles of leadership for restructuring his military teams for the complex battles in Iraq: shared consciousness and empowered execution. These principles have since become leadership principles for other complex environments.

> » **Shared consciousness:** The team is transparent in processes and functions so that members are equally knowledgeable and committed to shared goals. They are trusted to make decisions working from the same information and objectives. Interestingly, this concept of shared consciousness follows the model of a shared mental model described in the TeamSTEPPS curriculum.

> » **Empowered execution:** This requires the leader to remove his or her direct control over team members, decentralizing power. Taking advantage of the team's shared consciousness allows members to be both proactive and reactive in taking action when necessary. Sufficient knowledge of the situational context (shared consciousness) is required for members to be empowered.

McChrystal's analogy to the type of leadership required in this environment is to be less of a chess master, controlling every move of the team, and more of a gardener, enabling the team members to grow.

To achieve the interdependent principles of shared consciousness and empowered execution, trust and a common purpose must be valued within the team.

For APPs leading leaders in complex and ever-changing health care systems, developing teams that function together with a shared consciousness and empowered execution will guide their future success. Returning to Mona in Case Study 2, she likely realizes that in directing an office for APPs, she will be working primarily with many administrators, physicians, and other APPs who are strong leaders, goal oriented, and skilled in leading their own teams. She will not be able to establish herself in authority over the top of other teams, and will likely need to work toward the shared consciousness by learning from others and distributing information back and forth to maintain an equal base of knowledge across the institution about APP utilization. In reaching that shared consciousness, she can imagine the leaders of APPs within departments empowered to make appropriate decisions related to their areas.

SUMMARY POINTS

1. As health care teams share leadership responsibilities, the APP is able to volunteer directional advice more than ever before. It is imperative that the APP leader find the voice to address issues and offer recommendations and insights. Team training is necessary to develop an organizational structure that establishes *clear communication processes*, engaging all team members while maintaining mutual respect. *Shared leadership* roles reflect this open and accurate exchange of information, evident by the team's ability to *monitor situations*, respond when necessary, and provide *mutual support* to individual needs of the team members.

2. A health care team develops over time; the leader guides the team through common stages. First, team members need to identify their roles, potentially leading to conflict if roles collide. As the leader steers the team forward, the team reaches a consensus in responsibilities and can function well, but likely is challenged to grow and change over time (summarized by the stages of forming, storming, norming, performing, and adjourning). An effective team will recognize its mission and tasks (knowledge), manage its actions (skills), and collectively work together (attitude). Focusing on personnel morale and self-efficacy rather than economic strategies and technology will maximize the team's organizational health. The APP leader gains the most from organizing and facilitating productive meetings of the team.

3. When the team finds itself in a more complex environment, the principles of shared consciousness and empowered execution equally functioning together will help the team respond nimbly and adapt as needed in the midst of unpredictable circumstances. The leader in this type of team fosters the growth of each member to act responsibly in advancing the team's goals rather than the leader controlling each movement.

REFERENCES

Burke, C. S., Stagl, K. C., Kelin, C., Goodwin, G. F., Salas, E., & Halpin, S. M. (2006). What type of leadership behaviors are functional in teams? A meta-analysis. *Leadership Quarterly, 17*, 288–307.

Essary, A. C., Green, E. P., & Gans, D. N. (2016). Compensation and production in family medicine by practice ownership. *Health Services Research and Managerial Epidemiology, 3*, 1–5. doi:10.1177/2333392815624111

Lencioni, P. (2012). *The advantage: Why organizational health trumps everything else in business*. San Francisco, CA: Jossey-Bass.

Manges, K., Scott-Cawiezell, J., & Ward, M. M. (2017). Maximizing team performance: The critical role of the nurse leader. *Nursing Forum, 52*(1), 21–29.

McChrystal, S., Collins, T., Silverman, D., & Fussell, C. (2015). *Team of teams: New rules of engagement for a complex world*. New York, NY: Penguin Random House.

Morgan, P., Everett, C., & Hing, E. (2015). Nursing practitioners, physician assistants, and physicians in community health centers, 2006-2010. *Healthcare, 3*, 102–107.

Morrison, G., Goldfarb, S., & Lanken, P. N. (2010). Team training of medical students in the 21st century: Would Flexner approve? *Academic Medicine, 85*(2), 254–259.

Salas, E., Almeida, S. A., Salisbury, M., King, H., Lazzara, E. H., Lyons, R., . . . McQuillan, R. (2009). What are the critical success factors for team training in health care? *Joint Commission Journal on Quality & Patient Safety, 35*(8), 398–405.

Sheppard, F., Williams, M., & Klein, V. R. (2013). TeamSTEPPS and patient safety in health care. *Journal of Healthcare Risk Management, 32*(3), 5–10. doi: 10.1002/jhrm.21099

TeamSTEPPS® 2.0. (2015). Instructor manual. Rockville, MD: Agency for Healthcare Research and Quality. Retrieved from https://www.ahrq.gov/teamstepps/instructor/contents.html

Tuckman, B. W., & Jensen, M. A. C. (1977). Stages of small-group development revisited. *Group & Organization Studies, 2*(4), 419–427.

Yukl, G. (2013). *Leadership in organizations* (8th ed., p. 417). Upper Saddle River, NJ: Pearson.

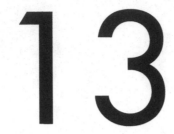

13

CLINICAL LEADER RESILIENCY AND BURNOUT

CRITICAL THINKING QUESTIONS

» What factors contribute to health care team stress and professional burnout?

» What can advanced practice providers (APPs) do to be more resilient and reduce their own risk of professional burnout?

» What can APP leaders do to reduce work–life stress in health care team members?

STRESSORS OF HEALTH CARE PROFESSIONALS

One of the greatest fears of any clinician in patient care is the specter of being sued for malpractice. There are stresses and measured risks in every line of work. In the medical community, lawsuits are common if not expected in some specialties of practice. Yet, when the call comes to inform the APP that a legal inquiry has begun, paralyzing doubts and dismay are uniform across all members of the profession. It is no surprise that the anxiety over malpractice threats is high on the list of reasons for professional burnout.

Other Factors Contributing to Stress

A healthy perspective that appreciates the risk of today's litigious environment carries the benefits of reminding the APP to maintain accurate documentation of health care records and communicate clearly with each patient.

Every individual has personal stress that is helpful in stimulating improved performance and motivating one toward healthy behaviors. However, factors causing stress accumulate, reaching a point when the burden of stress is deleterious. Of the many factors associated with stress in the professional role of APPs, several are unique to an individual practice setting; others are uniform across all APP work environments. Factors contributing to an APP's stress that cross health care delivery systems include:

» Expanding medical knowledge

» Increased productivity expectations

» Clerical burden of electronic health records (EHRs)

» Frequent medication reconciliation interruptions based on electronic prescriptions usage

» Greater insurance network requirements

» Changes in health care legislation

» Persistent risk of malpractice requiring excessive safeguards

» Tighter regulatory standards of meaningful use

» Onerous maintenance of certification or other credentialing requirements

The Endpoint of Excessive Stress: Burnout

Stressful periods for APPs are inevitable; waves of increased stress that then subside are expected. However, the unprecedented levels in health care performance expectations, accompanied by required scrutiny of clinical decision making, quality metrics, patient satisfaction scores, and cost measures maintain persistent stress. When stress is overwhelming without end in sight, burnout occurs.

Burnout, first described by Freudenberger (1974), is a syndrome with three main symptoms:

1. Emotional exhaustion

2. Depersonalization

3. Decreased work performance (see Table 13.1)

More common in those whose professional work require intense interrelationships with others, higher rates of burnout occur among teachers, social workers, police officers, and health care workers.

TABLE 13.1 Three Symptoms of Burnout

Symptom of Burnout	Description	Evident in Work	Quote Representing Symptom
Emotional exhaustion	Emotional energy is low	Fatigue, unexpected errors	*I can't keep going like this.*
Depersonalization	Sense of personal value is low	Absenteeism, loss of compassion	*What I do doesn't really matter.*
Low work performance	Productivity is decreased	Slow, careless	*I used to be able to do much more than now.*

Measures of burnout are established (e.g., Maslach, Jackson, & Leiter, 1996), but baselines are only now being established with little to compare. In a 2012 study of 7,288 U.S. physicians across all specialties, 45% reported at least one of the three symptoms of burnout. Estimates suggest burnout is over 50% among practicing U.S. physicians today (Shanafelt et al., 2012).

Levels of stress, depression, and medical symptoms were studied in 386 health professions students at one East Coast institution that compared medical, physician assistant (PA), and undergraduate nursing students. The results suggested that nursing students reported the least amount of stress and depression and the medical students reported the most, with the PA students in the middle (Hernandez, Blavo, Hardigan, Perez, & Hage, 2010). This study suggests there are varying levels of stress and depression between students in different health professions. Accurate measures of burnout encompassing the broad spectrum of APPs are not yet available.

A study of the effect of EHRs in medical practice offers an example of the stress induced by this technology designed to enhance medical informatics (Sinsky et al., 2016). Fifty-seven physicians from four states (Illinois, New Hampshire, Virginia, and Washington) were participants in the research, representing four specialties (family medicine, internal medicine, cardiology, and orthopedics). Four physician activities were measured by direct observation totaling 430 hours: (a) direct clinical face time with patients, (b) EHR deskwork, (c) administrative tasks, and (d) other tasks. Results showed that physicians spent 27% of their time in direct clinical face time with patients compared to 37% on EHR deskwork and 12% on other administrative tasks.

This study is limited due to the researchers selecting physicians who were notable as engaged in high-performing practices, so these results are not generalizable to other settings. However, the conclusions of this study showed that for every hour these physicians provided direct patient care, nearly 2 additional hours were spent on EHR deskwork and administrative tasks. There are no data available to compare with the era before EHRs regarding administrative tasks and documentation systems, such as time spent in handwriting chart notes; dictation and review; filling out test and treatment orders; and locating paper records, x-rays, and lab results.

Two of the factors of burnout, depersonalization and low work performance, directly relate to the outcomes of this study, contributing to the cynicism voiced by many about EHRs being associated with unwanted changes in the task of documentation in health care.

Outcomes of Burnout

The highest physician specialties facing burnout are critical care, urology, and emergency medicine, followed by family medicine and general internal medicine (Peckham, 2016). Among the primary care disciplines, this high rate of burnout in family medicine and general internal medicine raises concerns of workforce shortages and access to care. Effective utilization of APPs is suggested as part of the solution to these concerns, but stress and burnout among these professionals are also at risk. Data are not available specific to APPs, but using research outcomes from physician populations (Shanafelt, Dyrbye, & West, 2017), results of burnout lead to the following:

» More self-reported errors

» Higher turnover

» Increased mortality in hospitalized patients

» Reduced time in the clinical care of patients

» Physician suicides

The evidence behind these results of burnout is from localized studies and raises serious questions about how widespread these results may be. The latter finding about the physician suicide rate is a wider, national concern, as this rate of physician suicide has been higher than in the general U.S. population for a number of years. The incidence of undiagnosed depression among physicians holds a positive correlation with the increased physician suicide rate. A study of 17 states found that while mental illness is an important comorbidity for physicians dying by suicide, there are low rates of antidepressant usage based on postmortem toxicology reports (Gold, Sen, & Schwenk, 2013). Other drugs such as antipsychotics, benzodiazepines, and barbiturates were measured at higher levels in these physicians than in the nonphysician population of suicides. This suggests that physicians who die by suicide may be undertreated for depression.

Adjustable Factors of Burnout

There are marketplace forces, federal policy, and established economic streams that cannot easily be changed to reduce stress and burnout among health professionals. However, there are a number of factors manageable at the local level. Intentional efforts from the health care institution, combined with efforts by the individual, can reduce stress and prevent burnout, such as:

- » Reducing excessive workload
- » Alleviating clinical burdens
- » Repairing inefficiencies in the practice environment
- » Regaining a reasonable level of control over the work environment
- » Integrating work–life issues in better balance
- » Rediscovering meaningful work

The rest of this chapter is devoted to addressing practical solutions that meet these goals. The APP is a change-force to help implement supportive processes that will benefit the physicians and the health care team. Working toward these goals, the APP is likely to gain personally from these efforts as well.

CASE STUDY 1

Franklin has worked with Melanie, his physician employer, for 10 years in a busy general internal medicine practice of two internists. Melanie started the practice with one of her medical school classmates in this mid-sized community. Divorced years ago, she now brags that she is "married to her career." Hired as a new PA graduate, Franklin enjoys this rewarding and growing practice.

The practice implemented an EHR system 4 years ago and while it worked well, it did not interface with the EHR software adopted by the community's two hospitals and the pharmacies in town. The practice has recently had to implement an expensive and time-intensive conversion to a new system.

While stressful, Franklin enjoys his work but has noticed a change in Melanie over the last 6 months. She has a more negative attitude about her clinical work. Some patients tell Franklin that Melanie complains a lot about "the system" and they miss the caring bedside manner she used to show. She falls behind so that patients wait an hour or longer after their scheduled appointment times to be seen.

Franklin did not give it much attention until a couple of recent events. First, over the past 2 weeks, he has called her at night on a couple of occasions and could tell she was drinking alone. The last time, he needed her to come up to the hospital to see a patient, but she admitted she could not because of her alcohol consumption that night.

Franklin respects Melanie, yet she seems to be growing more distant from him. Their occasional lunch breaks together do not happen anymore. Yesterday she asked him to do evening rounds on a couple of her admitted patients so she could finish up at the clinic, a common request. However, she would usually give him detailed handoff information. This time she said, "Do whatever you wish; I'm sure they'll be fine."

He did not know what it was, but something was wrong.

HOW TO ADDRESS BURNOUT

In Case Study 1, Franklin thankfully recognizes early signs of burnout in the physician on his team. While there may be other explanations for Melanie distancing herself from him and her patients, he sees warning signs of burnout that deserve attention. Before initiating a conversation with her to explore his concerns, Franklin will be better equipped if he is more familiar with how to address issues of burnout.

The bleak path toward burnout can appear hopeless from the perspective of the strained individual, but many helpful options are available. The health care institution plays a key role in correcting physician burnout. As reported by the president and CEO of Mayo Clinic in Minnesota, many health care organizations erroneously believe professional satisfaction and burnout are the sole responsibility of the individual (Shanafelt & Noseworthy, 2017). However, the Mayo Clinic asserts that to support patient safety, avoid physician turnover, and sustain patient satisfaction, the health care organization is responsible for maintaining an environment of collaborative and productive health care teams. To this end, leaders of health care systems (e.g., health care executives, community boards, and private owners) must invest in supporting a committed professional workforce by intentional engagement, creating a culture that fosters vigor, dedication, and a balanced integration of work–life responsibilities.

The APP is often able to notice signs of burnout in physicians sooner than others are. The APP leader should be alert and responsive to act on any indications that suggest a physician is becoming overwhelmed with stress or dealing with depression or other mental health issues. Knowing what resources are available and, more importantly, engaging the team member (physician or other health professional) together with those resources may be among the most significant roles of the APP leader.

To be effective, it is imperative to combine a discussion of available resources with personal accountability and engagement by the individual; a coordinated effort is required (West, Dyrbye, Erwin, & Shanafelt, 2016). The APP leader has a clear opportunity to work toward this end.

FINDING RESILIENCY

Resilience is defined in many ways, but involves two attributes (Coutu, 2015):

» The ability to find meaning in the midst of difficulties

» The ability to improvise and function with what is available

Organizations and individuals who together demonstrate these attributes of resiliency will hold strong against the burden of stress and prevent burnout.

Organizational Interventions

As health care organizations implement processes to build resiliency and dissuade trends toward burnout, indicators to measure the success of their efforts are necessary. Adding measures of health care engagement and well-being of personnel alongside the quality performance metrics are suggested (Linzer et al., 2013). Current health care system metrics typically address the *Triple Aim*—enhancing patient experience, improving population health, and reducing costs (Berwick, Nolan, & Whittington, 2008). The design of these three dimensions of health care delivery optimizes health system performance. The Triple Aim, introduced nationally just prior to the recent U.S. health care reform, continues to be widely endorsed. A fourth proposed aim adds the goal of improved work–life of health care providers (Bodenheimer & Sinsky, 2014). Adding this metric to address the well-being of the providers creates the Quadruple Aim, proposed as a more meaningful and sustainable directive of health care delivery.

EXPLORE INCREASED UTILIZATION OF APPS

Adding APPs to the team is part of the solution when facing the challenges of high-volume patient workloads. For example, a study of PAs added to the staff of a surgical residency program showed that the addition of these APPs brought a measurable decrease in the residents' work hours and improved residents' work outlook over 6 months (Victorino & Organ, 2003). By adding one PA to each of four different surgical services, reduced work hours averaged 15 fewer hours per week over 6 months for the 10 to 12 surgery residents across all services. At the beginning of the study, 44% of the residents reported that the addition of PAs improved morale; within 6 months, this percentage was raised to 60%.

IMPROVE EHR DOCUMENTATION PROCESSES

Streamlining processes fosters resilient systems and reduces the burden of documentation of the clinical encounter. EHR methods to meet billing needs, quality reporting, and justification of tests do not project resiliency unless they are adaptable to distinct organizational applications. Some argue that today's current EHR demands are "unsustainable" (Shanafelt et al., 2017). Improvements to documentation methods should include input from the health care providers to evaluate their implications. Additional scheduled time for these administrative tasks may be necessary, or the team may redistribute and share the responsibilities for meeting EHR and administrative requirements (Linzer et al., 2013) by the addition of other staff.

IMPLEMENT A PROCESS IMPROVEMENT PROGRAM

To fully explore the scope of the problem within a health care organization, build resiliency, and target the right solutions for the local environment, a system-wide evaluation may be necessary. Formal programs are available, such as the Six Sigma process improvement methodology. Six Sigma offers proprietary consultants to evaluate management philosophies and develop a data-driven strategy to eliminate defects in dysfunctional organizational processes. Their management system depends on a five-step model of DMAIC, with successful applications in a variety of medical settings (e.g., Cima et al., 2011; Momani, Hirzallah, & Mumani, 2017).

» **Define**: Identifying the issues involved

» **Measure**: Using data points to identify inconsistencies or inaccuracies in the process

» **Analyze**: Based on data review and root-cause analysis, exploring and determining potential solutions

» **Improve**: Implementing improvement processes after sufficient planning and training

» **Control**: Assessing the quality of the improvements to determine long-term sustainability

Six Sigma is but one example of available models for an organized and thoughtful approach to determine improvements at an institutional level. The APP leader should take the opportunity to explore the potential benefits of a system-wide evaluation if a significant change is necessary across an institution.

REDUCE THE STIGMA OF MENTAL HEALTH DISORDERS AMONG PROFESSIONALS

At a higher level of the regulatory system, state licensing boards should review processes when inquiring about mental health conditions diagnosed in licensed providers. The lack of self-reporting depressive or anxiety disorders among physicians has been associated with concerns over the impact such reports would make on licensing decisions and renewals. Under-reporting these conditions leads to under-treatment, preventing those physicians who most need help from receiving appropriate care.

These suggested areas of focus to enhance the health care environment and lessen the risk of burnout are summarized in Table 13.2, along with additional ideas for health care systems to explore in gaining a more resilient organization. APP leaders should explore recommendations fitting their local setting to support the well-being of health care professionals in their institutions.

TABLE 13.2 Areas of Focus to Enhance the Health Care Environment for Providers

Area of Focus	Examples
Assess health care engagement and well-being of providers	Add one to three simple measures to existing quality performance metrics: • Control of work decisions • Time and pace of work • Provider satisfaction • Intent to leave practice • Alignment of organization values with provider • Benefits of work environment • Balance of work-life integration • Effectiveness of teamwork

(Continued)

TABLE 13.2 Areas of Focus to Enhance the Health Care Environment for Providers (*Continued*)

Area of Focus	Examples
Explore increased utilization of APPs	• Maximize current APPs' functions by assuring they are able to practice at the top of their license • Consider the effect of an additional APP in redistributing workloads while effectively adding productivity for the health care team
Improve EHR documentation processes	• Obtain input from providers to evaluate documentation methods • Schedule time for EHR and administrative tasks • Redistribute EHR and administrative requirements • Consider dictation/transcription processes that streamline provider communications
Improve efficiencies in the practice environment	• Examine need for system-wide evaluation of processes • Use a process improvement program to determine best solutions for unique needs of institution • Delegate or reduce clerical work
Reduce stigma of mental health disorders among professionals	• Develop support systems to help providers with mental health conditions to implement effective treatment • For providers with mental health needs, minimize risks to employment and professional career
Improve prior-authorization processes	• Work with insurance companies to standardize pre-approval requirements • Streamline institutional processes so that trained staff can manage prior-authorizations from routine EHR documentation • Minimize role of provider in managing administrative requirements once treatment/referral orders are determined
Modernize and align continuing medical education (CME) with certification and credentialing requirements	• Call for and participate in review processes that bring pertinent CME to align with professional certification and credentialing requirements • Remove requirements that are not relevant with clinical practice standards

APPs, advanced practice providers; EHR, electronic health record.

Personal Interventions

Personal resilience does not happen intuitively; it takes intentional focus. A study including interviews with 200 physicians of different ages and from different disciplines across Germany revealed three domains representing the prototypical development of personal resiliency (Zwack & Schweitzer, 2013):

» Finding gratification from therapeutic successes with patients

» Engaging in leisure activities, limiting work hours, and maintaining professional development

» Accepting personal and professional boundaries, maintaining an awareness of positive aspects of work

In applying these strategies of personal resilience, it is the professional responsibility of APPs to take care of themselves. Any standard of professionalism requires an honest, regular pattern of self-calibration. That said, it is not easy to recognize and respond to personal needs in the midst of challenging and stressful environments. The APP leader should be mindful of team members' behaviors and be prepared to recommend personal improvements to any individual within his or her circle of influence.

CASE STUDY 1 (CONTINUED)

Franklin cared about Melanie and knew that something was amiss. He asked if he could speak with her at the end of the day over coffee and she agreed.

"I respect the way you manage your patients and I continue to learn much from you," Franklin started after they sat down at a local coffee shop. "I think you're a fair employer and the way you support me as a PA has been great." He paused, struggling a bit with the next words. "It feels like something has changed, and I'm concerned about you. Can we talk about it? I'm wondering if you still enjoy your medical practice."

Melanie was willing to talk and appreciated Franklin's concern. She admitted that she was having some personal financial issues that were distracting her, and that yes, she was finding the burdens of the practice to be too much. She said, "It's just not enjoyable anymore."

"Let's consider the basics," Franklin said. "Are you sleeping okay?"

"Since you asked, I don't sleep great. I wake up, and more often my mind kicks in and sleep is all over."

"Thanks for being honest. How are you eating?" Franklin continued.

Melanie laughed. "I'm not your patient; you don't need to quiz me like one. But I'm eating fine, thanks."

Sipping his coffee, Franklin gave an embarrassed smiled. "Fair enough, though you would ask me the same things. You don't have to answer if you'd rather not, but we've known each other a long time. Can I ask you about your alcohol use? Is it any problem?"

"I've always been honest with you, Franklin." She seemed to appreciate his concern. "So with drinking, I might be doing a little more than I used to, but I'm not overdoing it. It just helps me relax in the evenings; that's all."

"Okay, that's all I needed to know," Franklin moved on. "Talk to me about the clinical practice. What is more of a problem for you now?"

"Of course, the EHR switch is a frustration for all of us. I don't think that's insurmountable—we'll get through it. I'm bothered by all the quality improvement demands at the hospitals. They've tightened their deadlines for my finishing up charts."

"You've always hated discharge notes," he joked sarcastically, smiling again. "Before EHR, you always had me dictating them for you."

"And now that I'm supposed to do my own in the EHR, they say it's easier but not in my book."

Franklin nodded, understanding.

"Then a couple weeks ago they told me my patient satisfaction scores were down compared to others. That hurts. I don't really understand it; maybe a couple people weren't very happy with me. That's why I asked you to do evening rounds yesterday. I knew our patients would be glad to see you. Anyway, administration said I must meet their benchmarks for patient satisfaction and the discharge documentation but didn't give me any ideas on what I should do differently."

"Thanks for telling me this, Melanie," Franklin could tell she was upset. "I know you better than those surveys. You're in a tough spot right now, and maybe your fatigue or personal stress is dragging you down. The patient satisfaction scores and the discharge summaries are both things we can fix. I can help if you want."

Melanie nodded. Franklin could see her eyes welling up.

"Let's work together on this. I have some ideas on getting the charts finished. Maybe you just need to set some personal goals; see about making some changes for improvement there. This isn't going to be that hard, Melanie."

From this short visit, Franklin was able to frame his realistic concerns that Melanie was facing burnout issues. She expressed poor sleep habits (emotionally exhausted), was cynical about her work (depersonalization), and had below-average quality indicators (low work performance), all three factors of the burnout syndrome. While her remark about financial issues was beyond him, her using alcohol as a means to relax at night suggested the possible start of an unhealthy dependency.

SELF-CARE

Each health care professional is personally responsible to take care of oneself, though encouragement from a trusted friend can help. In addition to seeing to one's own needs, the APP leader does well to support others toward healthy habits. The scenario in Case Study 1 is an example of what could be said, but every situation is unique and requires a thoughtful approach. Addressing issues of self-care include practicing healthy habits, utilizing personal strengths, and growing personal resiliency.

> » **Practicing healthy habits:** The APP must be self-aware of personal sleep hygiene, regular exercise, a balanced diet, and individual medical needs. Developing professional and personal relationships that stimulate individual growth and give perspective to life situations is in one's own control. There is no place for alcohol abuse, other substance abuse, or inappropriate sexual relationships. Particularly when life is challenging, exploring activities in the out-of-doors or volunteering to help others who have more severe needs can be restorative.
>
> APPs are individually responsible for identifying these personal priorities and taking deliberate steps to balance their personal and professional lives. The APP's professional relationship with members of the health care team brings opportunities to remind others of their own personal responsibility for healthy habits.
>
> » **Utilizing personal strengths:** In defining meaning and purpose with work, knowing one's strengths is helpful. Exercising those strengths affirms the individual and brings greater personal satisfaction. Among other available resources, the Gallup organization's StrengthFinders 2.0 web-based program is a well-recognized survey that helps a person explore his or her own talents and self-recognize areas that bring greater satisfaction. Based on their global client database, only 32% of those surveyed in the United States have the opportunity to do what they do best every day (Rath & Conchie, 2008). When an individual is self-aware of her or his strengths, working from these talents will optimize personal contributions to the workplace and reduce frustrations.
>
> Individual strengths vary from person to person. StrengthFinders 2.0 categorizes leadership strengths under four domains: executing, influencing, relationship building, and strategic thinking. APP leaders should note that an effective team has representation of strengths from each of these domains (Rath & Conchie, 2008).
>
> This is one method of determining one's strengths. Organizations may provide resources to identify personnel strengths and characteristics to help develop resilience and highly functioning teams, but the

individual must commit to the self-exploration and does not need to rely on the organization to provide the means.

» **Growing personal resiliency:** Personal resiliency comes from self-awareness based on significant personal reflection. Personal resiliency depends on one's own mindset when faced with challenges and crises. Handling the experience and bouncing back afterward is the best teacher of resiliency. Those with a tolerance for ambiguity likely fare better when times are uncertain or difficult. Ambiguity tolerance avoids finding circumstances as threatening or overwhelming. A fight-or-flight response is not expected when faced with obstacles. With a high tolerance for ambiguity, the individual is able to do more than just survive the uneasiness of uncertainty. Recognizing the discomfort as expected rather than a surprise, the individual is able to perform well and continue forward progress in spite of the unknown. This has been termed "nimbleness" (Conner, 1998) and considered a hallmark of resiliency. In fact, the nimble team is most productive in the midst of chaos, when it feels like the organization is about to fall apart or explode. The leader with the capacity to lead a team forward at that tipping point of the organization is effective likely due to a high tolerance for ambiguity.

This personal resiliency is best learned in the midst of trials. Prerequisites to growing resiliency are adopting healthy habits and utilizing one's strengths. These can be fostered by personal disciplines of mindfulness. Another exercise of mindfulness is the medical narrative, explored in Exercise 13.1.

EXERCISE 13.1 THE MEDICAL NARRATIVE

Narrative-based medicine was created to emphasize the experience of caring for patients from the science and objectivity of evidence-based medicine (Kalitzkus & Matthiessen, 2009). It is a therapeutic tool to enhance self-awareness, built on writing about a patient experience that caused the clinician to feel vulnerable or experience suffering. It may reflect the clinician's own experience as a patient, or an experience where the clinician was caring for a patient at a particularly difficult or challenging time. It requires the practice of mindfulness as the clinician must embody the experience to be able to write about it. Optional guidelines here may assist the writer in framing the exercise:

1. *Address the story to a specific person, whether it is actually read by that person or not. This helps the writer "tell the story" and often brings reflection on how best to phrase elements of the story.*

2. *Be specific in reporting what the clinician felt and experienced.*

3. *The writer determines the essential, relevant content. Details regarding the diagnostic science or therapeutic modalities are not required or expected.*

4. *Write the story as if living out the experience, rather than reporting knowledge about the experience.*

The process of writing the medical narrative itself is the therapy. This can serve as a weekly or daily exercise for the clinician. Reviewing the writings later brings further insights, exploring phrases that appear in multiple narratives. A recurrent feeling or emotion found in multiple narratives brings additional insight to the writer about meaningful perceptions.

LEADERSHIP IN PREVENTING BURNOUT

The health professional is typically attentive to detail, thinks critically, and derives decisions based on evidence. A team full of these personalities brings challenges to leadership due to the strengths of the personalities involved. The leader's additional role in helping the team explore ways to reduce stress can raise rather than lower anxiety.

A participatory leadership style is desirable when helping a team manage stress, inviting team members to contribute to leadership decisions (Shanafelt et al., 2017). Members need to be kept informed and have opportunities to make suggestions. The APP leader should facilitate, not force, professional development and acknowledge the work accomplished. This is best accomplished by finding aspects of work that are most rewarding for each team member and then focus on those aspects engaging members in activities that reflect their strengths, using coaching and mentoring methods.

SUMMARY POINTS

1. There are a number of factors beyond the control of the APP that contribute to the stress of health care systems, such as productivity expectations, EHR burdens, lawsuit risks, and insurance requirements, among others. However, many other factors of stress can be influenced by the APP to reduce the risk of burnout. These include efforts toward balancing clinician workloads, developing more efficient processes, creating more opportunities for meaningful work, and achieving improved integration of work–life balance.

2. Growth in the APP's personal management of stress occurs by becoming more resilient. Resiliency is the ability to find meaning in difficult times, effectively moving forward despite the challenges. Physicians report that the keys to resiliency are finding meaning in the care of patients, alongside establishing work–life boundaries by limiting work hours and making time for leisure activities. The APP should be mindful of these values and be devoted to healthy habits, working out of one's strengths to become more resilient.

3. The APP leader should be vigilant in observing behaviors among the health care team that manifest emotional exhaustion, depersonalization (cynicism), or low performance metrics. Each of these would indicate concerns of burnout but be ignored by the individual until the APP asks. By modeling the practice of self-care, the APP gains credibility to spur team members in positive attitudes and health habits. The APP leader may make recommendations to the administration on ways to streamline EHR processes, improve efficiencies, and build community, all reducing stress factors. Adding a measure of employee well-being to the existing performance measures may prove beneficial to identify what gains are achieved.

REFERENCES

Berwick, D. M., Nolan, T. W., & Whittington, J. (2008). The triple aim: Health, care, and cost. *Health Affairs, 27*(3), 759–769.

Bodenheimer, T., & Sinsky, C. (2014). From triple aim to quadruple aim: Care of the patient requires care of the provider. *Annals of Family Medicine, 12*(6), 573–576.

Cima, R. R., Brown, M. J., Hebl, J. R., Moore, R., Rogers, J. C., Kollengode, A., . . . Deschamps, C. (2011). Use of lean and Six Sigma methodology to improve operating room efficiency in a high-volume tertiary-care academic medical center. *Journal of the American College of Surgeons, 213*, 83–92.

Conner, D. R. (1998). *Leading at the edge of chaos: How to create a nimble organization.* New York, NY: Wiley.

Coutu, D. (2015). How resilience works. In Harvard Business Review, *HBR's 10 must reads: On emotional intelligence* (pp. 105–118). Boston, MA: Harvard Business Review Press.

Freudenberger, H. J. (1974). Staff burn-out. *Journals of Social Issues, 30*(1), 159–165.

Gold, K. J., Sen, A., & Schwenk, T. L. (2013). Details on suicide among US physicians: Data from the National Violent Death Reporting System. *General Hospital Psychiatry, 35*(1), 45–49.

Hernandez, M. B., Blavo, C., Hardigan, P. C., Perez, A. M., & Hage, K. (2010). Differences in perceived stress, depression, and medical symptoms among medical, nursing, and physician assistant students: A latent class analysis. *Annals of Behavioral Science and Medical Education, 16*(1), 35–39. doi:10.1007/BF03355116

Kalitzkus, V., & Matthiessen, P. F. (2009). Narrative-based medicine: Potential, pitfalls, and practice. *Permanente Journal, 13*(1), 80–86.

Linzer, M., Levine, R., Meltzer, D., Poplau, S., Warde, C., & West, C. P. (2013). 10 bold steps to prevent burnout in general internal medicine. *Journal of General Internal Medicine, 29*(1), 18–20. doi:10.1007/s11606-013-2597-8

Maslach, C., Jackson, S. E., & Leiter, M. P. (1996). *Maslach Burnout Inventory Manual* (3rd ed). Palo Alto, CA: Consulting Psychologists Press.

Momani, A., Hirzallah, M., & Mumani, A. (2017). Improving employee's safety awareness in healthcare organizations using the DMAIC quality improvement approach. *Journal for Healthcare Quality, 39*(1), 54–63.

Peckham, C. (2016). Medscape lifestyle report 2016: Bias and burnout. Retrieved from http://www.medscape.com/features/slideshow/lifestyle/2016/public/overview#page=1

Rath, T., & Conchie, B. (2008). *Strengths-based leadership.*, New York, NY: Gallup Press.

Shanafelt, T. D., Boone S., Tan L., Dyrbye, L. N., Sotile W., Satele, D., . . . Oreskovich, W. R. (2012). Burnout and satisfaction with work–life balance among U.S. physicians compared to the general U.S. population. *Annals of Internal Medicine, 172*(18), 1377–1385.

Shanafelt, T. D., Dyrbye, L. N., & West, C. P. (2017). Addressing physician burnout: The way forward. *Journal of the American Medical Association, 317*(9), 901–902. doi:10.1001/jama.2017.0076

Shanafelt, T. D., & Noseworthy, J. H. (2017). Executive leadership and physician well-being: Nine organizational strategies to promote engagement and reduce burnout. *Mayo Clinic Proceedings, 92*(1), 129–146. doi:10.1016/j.mayocp.2016.10.004

Sinsky, C., Colligan, L., Li, L., Prgomet, M., Reynolds, S., Goeders, L., . . . Blike, G. (2016). Allocation of physician time in ambulatory practice: A time and motion study in 4 specialties. *Annals of Internal Medicine, 165*(11), 753–760. doi:10.7326/M16-0961

Victorino, G. P., & Organ, C. H. Jr. (2003). Physician assistant influence on surgery residents. *Archives of Surgery, 138*, 971–976.

West, C. P., Dyrbye, L. N., Erwin, P. J., & Shanafelt, T. D. (2016). Interventions to prevent and reduce physician burnout: A systematic review and meta-analysis. *Lancet, 388*, 2272–2281.

Zwack, J., & Schweitzer, J. (2013). If every fifth physician is affected by burnout, what about the other four? Resilience strategies of experienced physicians. *Academic Medicine, 88*(3), 382–389.

PART 4
Looking Ahead

14

LEADING INTO THE FUTURE

CRITICAL THINKING QUESTIONS

» **What trends are notable in the evolution of health care that can be influenced by advanced practice provider (APP) leaders?**

» **What leadership strategies are effective in guiding health care teams when the future is uncertain?**

Try to balance the handle of a broomstick in the open palm of the hand, the broom bristles pointing to the sky. It is nearly impossible to keep it upright if the holder attends to watching only the palm of the hand to make adjustments in balance. The actual control is in the palm responding to the sway of the broom as it leans one way and then the other. But this is not where the eyes should focus.

As soon as the holder gazes up to the top of the broom, where the broom head is aiming, the ability to balance the broom is much easier. Watching the top of the broom head indicates the needed adjustments. The hand still moves to balance the tip of the handle resting in the palm, now guided by what is happening on the other end of the broom. So too, it is best for the leader to focus on what is ahead of the team to guide the direction.

THE FUTURE OF HEALTH CARE DELIVERY

Revelations of what is coming in health care are predictable by scanning the trends of current markets and industries. Directly effecting health care, trends with no indication of slowing include:

» Greater automation

» Increasing immediate information access

» More highly specialized and individually specific advanced technologies

CASE STUDY 1

John is the 55-year-old African American male with chest pain and EKG findings of an acute inferior wall myocardial infarction introduced in Case Study 1 in Chapter 2. He has agreed to follow his nurse practitioner's (NP's) recommendation (Pam) to be transferred from her clinic immediately to Central Community Hospital Emergency Room (ER). With the emergency unit already dispatched, Pam, as promised, has been in contact with the ER staff. In a matter of seconds, John is loaded by gurney into the mobile unit.

"How is your chest pain now, John?" the paramedic asks as they drive away from the clinic. "We can give you something more for the pain."

"It's better, maybe just a 3 on your scale now," John responds, "but the nausea is worse—I feel lightheaded."

The paramedic gestures to his right side, "Here's Orlanzo, one of the physician assistants (PAs) at Central Community Hospital." The paramedic addresses a translucent image that suddenly appears inside the vehicle. "Orlanzo, this is John. His pain is down to a 3, but his nausea is worse. I know you've got his vital signs."

John sees Orlanzo, but also sees right through him. He's a projected image. Orlanzo immediately addresses John.

"Nice to meet you, John. Don't mind my holographic image here; I'll be with you in the flesh as soon as you get here. Pam has told me all about you, and I know you aren't crazy about coming here. You're doing the right thing and we're going to do our best for you. Let's get your nausea under control." Despite the translucent form, John is relieved to see and hear this reassurance. He closes his eyes, hearing Orlanzo talking to the paramedic.

". . . and let's raise this to a level 6 transport," Orlanzo says to the paramedic. "We need to get John here as soon as possible."

The paramedic pushes a button on the vehicle and the driverless mobile unit zooms through the streets with all intersections and lights coordinated to clear traffic, redirecting all other driverless vehicles. With travel time cut in half, John has a smooth and fast transport.

Case Study 1 presents a different patient care system than anticipated from its presentation in Chapter 2. The futuristic environment of this scenario has Orlanzo serving as an APP in completely different surroundings than today. However, the skills needed for leading patient care and his health care team remain the same.

Whatever may be the future of health care delivery, this example suggests that the principles of clinical leadership will not change. In the future, Pam will still be faced with patients who, because they misunderstand or are obstinate, need to be persuaded to make wise decisions for their health care. APPs will still need strong communication skills when working in health care teams. The health care environment will continue to face uncertainty and change, requiring the APP to help the team stay nimble, adapting to the needs. Opportunities to influence the team will remain prominent; the APP will be sought to lead. Perhaps the most important decision for the APP is to decide if he or she will step up to the call.

IMMEDIATE FUTURE OF HEALTH CARE SYSTEMS

There are expectations for the near future that are clearly imminent. Due to market forces and the current direction of governmental policies, health care practices traditionally owned and managed by physicians are fading due to challenges in profitability. Large group practices and hospitals with expanded administrative teams are scaled by size and patient volume to better manage the breadth and depth of bureaucracy and regulatory requirements. The days of solo or small group physician-owned practices are waning, replaced by practices owned by larger groups and hospitals. As evidence for this trend, in the early 1980s, 40% of physicians were in solo practices compared to 20% in 2014, according to the AMA Physician Practice Benchmark Surveys (Kane 2015). The number of physicians employed by hospital-owned practices has increased 230% in the past four years (Baker, Bundorf, Devlin, & Kessler, 2016).

Factors contributing to this shift that are not likely to change are the further expansion of electronic health record (EHR) applications, reimbursement policies, and meaningful use requirements. Larger practices and hospitals cost-effectively manage the financial and administrative challenges associated with these technologies and regulations. The Medicare value-based payment incentives are examples of processes implemented more effectively by larger group practices and hospitals with the benefit of greater financial viability.

APPs in states that are dependent on physician supervision may find the shift away from physician-owned practices will influence APP employment. The benefit the APP brings to the practice is shifting to the organizations, hospitals, and large group practices. The measure of this effect is not clear and APP leaders must stay vigilant to demonstrate the contributions of APPs.

TABLE 14.1 Distinguishing Characteristics of Where Humans and Technology Excel

Where Humans Excel	Where Technology Excels
Imagination	Location of resources
Compassion	Mechanical learning
Altruism	Independent processing
Common sense	Pattern recognition
Support of virtues	Classification of massive data
Hope	Predictable accuracy
Abstract learning	Tireless continuous function

THE HUMAN COMPONENT IN LEADERSHIP

EHR and technological advancements are expected only to increase with improved applications and utilization that is more widespread. In the midst of this ever-greater reliance on technology, the human component of health care cannot be diminished. Personal qualities that distinguish humans from machines (see Table 14.1) are particularly welcome in people-oriented services such as patient care. Characteristics exercised by the APP contribute to health care delivery in ways technology never will, in areas such as altruism, virtues, and imagination.

Humans will also remain fallible. With the human propensity for error, APPs should pursue application of technologies that will help prevent mistakes. Leaders will guide the effective utilization of technology by advancing health care that is safer, more accurate, and more useful.

The human component should consistently accompany technology in health care delivery. In leading health care teams and direct patient care, highly complex or invasive technology requires APPs to lead an increase in uniquely human traits, such as providing greater levels of compassion, common sense, and hope.

OUTCOMES OF EFFECTIVE CLINICAL LEADERSHIP

While health care system change is inevitable, the goals of effective leadership are the same. The Center for Creative Leadership (CCL), a nonprofit educational institute that offers leadership development consulting services across the world (Van Velsor, McCauley, & Ruderman, 2010), developed an optimal framework for highly functioning health care organizations. Based on its study of leadership research, direct involvement with over 400 various health service organizations and leadership development with thousands of health care leaders, CCL reports seven key characteristics of best-practice organizational capacity in high-performing hospitals and health care systems (Browning, Torain, & Patterson, 2011):

» Clinical staff members at all levels are engaged in work by clear, direct, open, and honest communication.

» Proactive collaboration is emphasized.

» Staff are recruited and retained to support care that is compassionate, safe, and of high quality.

» Innovative processes function throughout the health care system.

» A culture of continuous learning is fostered.

» In times of ambiguity, leaders guide the team to act strategically and decisively.

» Employees are supported to manage stress and enjoy healthy relationships.

These characteristics reflect a health care organization that is able to thrive in the midst of challenges. Together, the characteristics are idealistic and challenging to attain and maintain in any environment. The APP leader who contributes to seeing these outcomes reached will foster an environment that achieves advancement in high-quality health care delivery.

LEADERSHIP CHARACTERISTICS FOR UNCERTAIN TIMES

Future trends suggest that the complexity, uncertainty, and occasional chaos common in health care systems today are not going away. In this unstable environment, some organizations fail and others thrive. Collins and Hansen (2011) studied U.S. companies that over 15 years were able to beat industry performance indexes a minimum of 10 times. In analyzing traits of those high-performing businesses compared to other companies, differences were not centered on vision casting, risk-taking, or creativity. Themes common to these top organizations were three-fold: being more disciplined, empirical, and paranoid. These themes require leadership action further defined as follows:

» **Fanatic discipline:** Avoiding any sense of bureaucratic control, this theme refers to leading a team to be relentlessly consistent in maintaining the values, goals, processes, and standards.

» **Empirical creativity:** Bold, innovative actions guided by the leader are supported by empirical evidence.

» **Productive paranoia:** This requires the leader to be vigilant, noting potential challenges, threats, and changes, especially when things are going well. The team considers worst-case scenarios by having contingency plans and work-arounds maintaining a margin of safety.

OUTCOMES OF EFFECTIVE LEADERSHIP

APPs, like all clinicians, seek to practice according to evidence-based principles of medicine. It will remain the challenge of APP leaders to pursue evidence-based leadership concepts that are effective in the local setting. The application of leadership remains dependent on the individual leader, the team members and the environment, all which carry unique influences. One cannot measure the level of leader success until after a project is completed. While success stories and recommendations abound, such as those creatively offered by Collins & Hansen, it falls on the leader to proactively and boldly step forth and lead.

The mistake is the belief that exceptional leadership outcomes occur by chance, that the winds blow as they will and that sometimes it works and sometimes it does not. The evidence shared throughout this text reminds us that adequate preparation for leadership is required, thoughtful leader actions are significant, and character and integrity often carry the day.

SUMMARY POINTS

1. There are expected trends in health care that are outside the influence of APPs, such as federal regulatory change. The movement away from physician-owned practices to hospital-owned practices and other large group practices is growing, which will have an unpredictable effect on APP employment, perhaps with benefits or challenges. Other trends such as increased utilization of EHRs and other diagnostic and therapeutic technologies present opportunities for APPs to guide future applications in support of high-quality patient care delivered by health care teams. Effective APP leadership can readily address the uniquely human characteristics within these advancements, such as health care teams exercising common sense and ensuring safety and patient care remaining virtuous and compassionate.

2. In light of the ambiguities of tomorrow's health care systems because of continued but unknown health care reform measures, APP leaders

need to act strategically and decisively. Effective leadership actions will maintain a discipline consistent with the values and standards of the organization. The leaders must be boldly creative based on thoughtful, evidence-based strategies and remain exceedingly vigilant to potential problems. Responses can then be made nimbly and proactively to stay the course of advancing improved health care outcomes.

REFERENCES

Baker, L. C., Bundorf, K. M., Devlin, A. M., & Kessler, D. P. (2016). Hospital ownership of physicians: Hospital versus physician perspectives. *Medical Care Research and Review,* 1–12. doi:10.1177/1077558716676018

Browning, H. W., Torain, D. J., & Patterson, T. E. (2011). *Collaborative health-care leadership: A six-part model for adapting and thriving during a time of transformative change,* White Paper (published 2011, reprinted 2016). Center for Creative Leadership. Retrieved from http://www .ccl.org/leadership/pdf/research/collaborativeHealthcareLeadership.pdf

Collins, J., & Hansen, M. T. (2011). *Great by choice.* New York, NY: Harper Collins.

Kane, C. K. (2015). *Updated data on physician practice arrangements: Inching toward hospital ownership.* Chicago, IL: American Medical Association.

Van Velsor, E., McCauley, C. D., & Ruderman, M. N. (2010). *The center for creative leadership handbook of leadership development.* San Francisco, CA: Jossey-Bass.

APPENDICES

APPENDICES

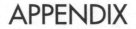

APPENDIX

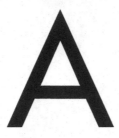

LEADER INTERVIEW ACTIVITY

The Leader Interview Activity introduces the student to a general inquiry about leadership principles and skills.

LEARNING OBJECTIVE

After completion of this assignment, the student will be able to stratify leader qualities and explore their origins.

LEARNER CONTENT AND DESIGN

The interview questions offer a framework to explore the following learner topics:

- » Self-assessment of leadership
- » Nature versus nurture of leadership
- » Leadership mentors
- » Leadership traits
- » Ineffective leadership
- » Measures of effective leadership
- » Leadership succession planning

The format of this assignment is tailored for online learning management systems (LMS). This promotes interaction between student peers as they each share their leader interviews with one another. The assignment can be modified to fit a classroom or paper-based activity if desired.

In this LMS format, the student posts the assignment for viewing and critique by student peers. A second assignment invites peers to share their feedback with the student–author of the interview summary. The focus of the feedback activity is to trigger the student to exercise learning in identifying and valuing leadership qualities in his or her peers' reports.

OPTIONAL MODIFICATIONS

1. The leader to be interviewed should be a member of a health care team.

2. The leader to be interviewed should be an advanced practice provider.

LEADER INTERVIEW ASSIGNMENT

1. Select a leader around you. You may self-define what "leader" means for the context of this assignment.

2. Interview that leader, including the following questions:

   a. Do you consider yourself a leader? Why or why not?

   b. Who in your experience has taught you the most about leadership? Please describe.

   c. What three principles are most important for being a good leader?

   d. Give a story of when your leadership was not effective enough and what you would change.

   e. Give a story of when your leadership contributed to a positive outcome.

   f. If you left your position tomorrow, how well would the group you lead fare?

   (Additional questions are welcome, though not required.)

3. From the information provided by this interview and any additional material you wish to contribute about the leader, write a one- or two-page (300–600 words) interview summary. Generously use quotes from the leader to describe his or her leadership qualities.

4. Post your interview summary on the Discussion Board.

Evaluation Criteria

The interview summary will be evaluated according to the following criteria:

» **Qualities:** The individual's qualities determining that he or she is a "leader" are clearly described.

» **Effectiveness:** The effectiveness of the leader by external outcomes is clearly described.

» **Challenges:** The challenges this person faces in being a good leader are presented.

» **Quotes:** At least five distinct quotes from the leader are used to support the content of the summary.

FEEDBACK ASSIGNMENT

1. Read at least one of your peers' interview summary postings.

2. Respond to the interview summary on the Discussion Board, answering the following three questions:

   a. Why did you like this particular leader?

   b. How does this leader compare to the leader you interviewed?

   c. What is the main attribute or characteristic that this leader possesses that contributes to successful leadership? Explain your answer.

3. The feedback is estimated to require at least 200 words to adequately address these questions. Please submit the feedback on the Discussion Board.

4. The feedback will be evaluated based on satisfactorily answering the above three questions.

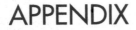

APPENDIX

B

MOVIE REPORT ON LEADERSHIP

The Movie Report on Leadership engages the student in observing active leadership characteristics and traits as seen in popular culture movies and measuring their effect on those around the leader.

LEARNING OBJECTIVE

After completion of this assignment, the student will be able to analyze leadership characteristics and traits as observed in action.

Prerequisite knowledge: The student should have reviewed at least Chapters 1 through 3 prior to this activity.

LEARNER CONTENT AND DESIGN

The movie report guides the student to explore the effectiveness of leadership and use of power and influence as exhibited in action. The balance of power and the degree of success of the leader provide qualitative measures for the student to assess the leadership outcomes.

The format of this assignment is tailored for online learning management systems (LMS). This promotes interaction between student peers as they each share their movie reports with one another. The assignment can be modified to fit a classroom or paper-based activity if desired.

In this LMS format, the student posts the assignment for viewing and critique by student peers. A second assignment invites peers to share their feedback with the student–author of the movie report. The focus of the feedback activity is to engage the student in the following:

1. Generate new influence tactics that may apply to leadership situations;

2. Compare different leadership traits in relation to those recognized in the leader character portrayed in the movie;

3. Analyze determinants of a successful leader.

OPTIONAL MODIFICATIONS

1. The setting of the movie should be primarily in a health care environment.

2. The leader studied in this report should be a health care professional involved in direct patient care.

MOVIE REPORT ON LEADERSHIP ASSIGNMENT

1. Select and watch a movie that features a leader.

2. Provide a narrative report, no longer than two pages (approximately 600 words), to address the following questions:

   a. What is the movie and who is the leader? Why did you select this leader?

   b. Discuss which two power types are primarily exercised by the leader and support your discussion with examples.

   c. How does the leader manage the balance of power (e.g., is power acquired or lost)? Provide examples.

   d. Discuss three influence tactics used by the leader and what their outcomes were. How well did the influence tactics work in achieving a desired outcome?

   e. Discuss the measure of this leader's success based on the response of those being led (e.g., are those being led committed, compliant, or resistant?).

   f What is your favorite "leadership" scene from the movie and why is it special?

3. The movie report should be posted on the Discussion Board.

Evaluation Criteria

The movie report will be evaluated according to the following criteria:

» **Power:** Two power types are adequately described.

» **Balance:** The balance of power is clearly addressed.

» **Influence:** Three influence tactics are adequately described.

» **Success:** The measure of success is defined.

» **Qualities:** A "favorite scene" is representative of leader qualities.

FEEDBACK ASSIGNMENT

1. Read at least one of your peers' movie reports.

2. Respond to the report on the Discussion Board answering the following four questions:

    a. What additional influence tactic would you recommend that this leader consider using and why?

    b. Based on the information in the report, what three character traits (e.g., honesty, attractiveness, selfishness) does this leader hold?

    c. What leadership style or trait does the leader/character in this movie best represent as described in this report? Explain your answer.

    d. Would you consider this leader successful? Explain your answer.

3. The feedback is estimated to require at least 300 words to adequately address these questions.

4. The feedback will be evaluated based on satisfactorily answering the four questions.

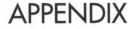

APPENDIX

C

HISTORICAL LEADER CHARACTERIZATION

The Historical Leader Characterization engages the student in identifying leadership attributes by studying historical records and experiences of a recognized leader of the past.

LEARNING OBJECTIVE

After completion of this assignment, the student will be able to explain leadership qualities and traits observed in past leaders.

Prerequisite knowledge: The student should have reviewed at least Chapters 2 through 4 prior to this activity.

LEARNER CONTENT AND DESIGN

The characterization report requires the student to find credible evidence of leadership and identify the qualities that contribute to the leadership outcomes. The leadership traits are explored in the context of what the student values and could apply to his or her own experience.

The format of this assignment is tailored for online learning management systems (LMS). This promotes interaction between student peers as they each share their characterizations with one another. The assignment can be modified to fit a classroom or paper-based activity if desired.

In this LMS format, the student posts the assignment for viewing and critique by student peers. A second assignment invites peers to share their feedback with the student–author of the historical leader characterization. The focus of the feedback activity is to engage the student in relating information learned about leadership to the characteristics and traits observed in or reported about the historical leader.

OPTIONAL MODIFICATIONS

1. The historical leader should be from past health care environments.

2. The historical leader selected should be an advanced practice provider.

HISTORICAL LEADER CHARACTERIZATION ASSIGNMENT

Select a historical leader who is no longer living and complete the following outline based on credible information about the leader.

A. **Leader Name:**

B. **Why did you select this leader** (Why should we read your characterization)?

C. **Chronology of leader events** (5–10 marks of training or experience that formed the leader):

1.

2.

3.

4.

5.

6.

7.

8.

9.

10.

D. **How has this leader influenced your own leadership** (include examples from your own life supporting your description of this influence)?

Evaluation Criteria

The historical leader characterization will be evaluated according to the following criteria:

- **Qualities:** The individual's qualities that determine he or she is a "leader" are clearly described.

- **Effectiveness:** The effectiveness of the leader by external outcomes is clearly described.

- **Development:** The process of leadership development is described by historical milestones.

- **Influence:** The leader has offered a clear influence to the student with specific examples cited.

- **Conciseness:** The assignment is limited to no more than two pages (600 words) of text.

FEEDBACK ASSIGNMENT

1. Read at least one of your peers' historical leader characterization postings.

2. Provide feedback to your peer's characterization on the Discussion Board by responding to these three statements:

   a. Discuss how your peer's characterization compares to one or more established leadership styles or traits. Provide citations for any resources used in your discussion.

   b. Among the seven power types described in Chapter 2, Power and Influence, describe at least two power types exhibited by your peer's historical leader characterization and support your answer.

   c. Discuss at least one aspect of the historical leader's qualities that might also apply to you in your own current or future leadership situations.

3. The feedback is estimated to require at least 250 words to adequately address these statements.

4. The feedback will be evaluated based on satisfactorily answering the three statements.

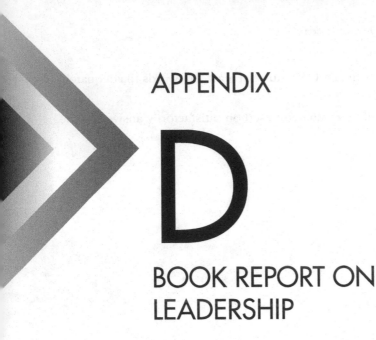

APPENDIX

D

BOOK REPORT ON LEADERSHIP

The Book Report on Leadership engages the student in studying leadership skills and behaviors in a self-selected, published book and applying what is learned to current, relevant leadership opportunities.

LEARNING OBJECTIVE

After completion of this assignment, the student will be able to analyze the application of leadership skills and behaviors.

Prerequisite knowledge: The student should have reviewed at least Chapters 2 to 5 prior to this activity.

LEARNER CONTENT AND DESIGN

The book report has the student confront relevant leadership concepts described in a self-selected text and explore in more detail the strengths and weaknesses of leadership from the student's own perspective. With the prerequisite learning acquired, the student is positioned to compare and contrast various leadership models from both the leader and the team's perspectives, and can draw conclusions from the book as they apply to the student's leadership arena.

The format of this assignment is tailored for online learning management systems (LMS). This promotes interaction between student peers as they each share their book reports with one another. The assignment can be modified to fit a classroom or paper-based activity if desired.

In this LMS format, the student posts the assignment for viewing and critique by student peers. A second assignment invites peers to share their own feedback with the student–author of the book report. The focus of the feedback activity is to engage the student in critically comparing information learned from the self-selected book with the alternative book as described by a student peer in the report. This both heightens the student's awareness of the self-selected book and broadens the student's understanding by comparisons with other leadership models.

Optional modifications: The instructor selects a single book or a shorter, more focused list of choices for the students.

BOOK REPORT ON LEADERSHIP ASSIGNMENT

1. Select a book from the list provided at the end of the assignment or other list provided by the instructor. After reading the book, submit a book report including the following elements:

   a. Brief overview of the book

   b. Favorite quote from the book with discussion of selection

   c. Application to clinical leadership of advanced practice providers (APPs)

   d. Rate the usefulness of this book to APP leaders (using a scale of 1 to 10, 10 being "best") including a discussion of your evidence in support of this rating

2. The book report should be no longer than two pages (approximately 600 words).

3. Post the book report as an attachment on the Discussion Board.

Evaluation Criteria

The book report will be evaluated according to the following criteria:

» **Summary:** The overview summarizes key principles of the book.

» **Favorite quote:** The "favorite quote" is clarified in the context of the book and why it is valued by the student.

» **Application:** Practical applications to APP leadership are clearly explored.

» **Rating:** Rating is supported by an objective and logical discussion.

FEEDBACK ASSIGNMENT

1. Read at least one of your peers' book reports.

2. Respond to the report on the Discussion Board by answering the following four questions:

   a. What did you particularly like about this book report in exploring leadership?

   b. How do the leader principles in the book compare to your expectations of your own leadership style as an APP?

   c. How does this book's rating compare to your own book rating? Please explain your answer.

   d. How likely are you to read this book? Please explain your answer.

3. The feedback is estimated to require at least 300 words to adequately address these questions.

4. The feedback will be evaluated based on satisfactorily answering the four questions.

SUGGESTED BOOK LIST

Select a book from the list below:

» *Great by Choice: Uncertainty, Chaos and Luck: Why Some Thrive Despite Them All*, J. Collins and M. T. Hansen, 2011.

» *Leading at the Edge of Chaos: How to Create a Nimble Organization*, D. Conner, 1998.

» *HBR's 10 Must Reads on Leadership, Harvard Business Review*, B. George, 2011.

» *Endurance: Shackleton's Incredible Voyage*, A. Lansing, 2007.

» *The Prince*, N. Machiavelli, 1513.

» *The 5 Levels of Leadership*, J. Maxwell, 2011.

» *Team of Teams*, S. McChrystal, 2015.

» *Strengths Based Leadership: Great Leaders, Teams and Why People Follow*, T. Rath and B. Conchie, 2009.

» *The Contrarian's Guide to Leadership*, S. Sample, 2002.

» *The Practitioner's Guide to Governance as Leadership*, C. A. Trower, 2013.

» *The Art of War*, S. Tzu, (5th century BCE).

» *Servant Leadership in Higher Education*, D. Wheeler, 2012.

» *Wooden on Leadership*, J. Wooden, 2005.

» Or other leadership book if approved by instructor.

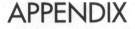

APPENDIX

E

CURRENT LEADER CHARACTERIZATION

The Current Leader Characterization engages the student in identifying clinical leadership attributes by studying a contemporary leader in health care today.

LEARNING OBJECTIVE

After completion of this assignment, the student will be able to evaluate leadership qualities, traits, and behaviors of current leaders in health care.

Prerequisite knowledge: The student should have reviewed at least Chapters 1 through 5 prior to this activity.

LEARNER CONTENT AND DESIGN

The characterization report requires the student to find credible evidence of leadership and evaluate the qualities that contribute to the leadership outcomes. The leadership traits and behaviors are explored in the context of what the student values in and could apply to his or her own experience.

The format of this assignment is tailored for online learning management systems (LMS). This promotes interaction between student peers as they each share their characterizations with one another. The assignment can be modified to fit a classroom or paper-based activity if desired.

In this LMS format, the student posts the assignment for viewing and critique by student peers. A second assignment invites peers to share their own feedback with the student–author of the current leader characterization. The focus of the feedback activity is to engage the student in relating information learned about leadership and followership to the qualities, traits, and behaviors observed in or reported about the health care leader.

Optional Modifications

1. The current leader may be selected from any environment, not limited to health care.
2. The current leader selected should be an advanced practice provider.

CURRENT LEADER CHARACTERIZATION ASSIGNMENT

Select a current leader in health care and complete the following outline based on credible information about the leader.

A. **Leader Name:**

B. **Why did you select this leader** (Why should we read your characterization)?

C. **Chronology of leader events** (5–10 marks of training or experience that formed the leader):

1.

2.

3.

4.

5.

6.

7.

8.

9.

10.

D. **Leadership Styles**

Using the leadership models, traits, and behaviors addressed thus far in this text, discuss at least three practical examples of how this leader fits a specific model, trait, or behavior (e.g., describe the leader's high-exchange and low-exchange member relationships, describe situations where the leader demonstrated transformational behaviors such as individualized consideration and intellectual stimulation). More than one model, trait, or behavior may be described.

E. **How has this leader influenced your own leadership** (include examples from your own life supporting your description of this influence)?

Evaluation Criteria

The current leader characterization will be evaluated according to the following criteria:

○ **Qualities:** The individual's qualities that determine he or she is a "leader" are clearly described.

○ **Effectiveness:** The effectiveness of the leader by external outcomes is clearly described.

○ **Development:** The process of leadership growth is described by developmental milestones.

○ **Leadership styles:** At least three examples are given related to specific leadership theories and traits.

○ **Influence:** The leader has offered a clear influence to the student with specific examples cited.

○ **Conciseness:** The assignment is limited to no more than three pages (900 words) of text.

FEEDBACK ASSIGNMENT

1. Read at least one of your peers' current leader characterization postings.

2. Provide feedback to your peer's characterization on the Discussion Board by responding to these four questions:

   a. Why did you like this particular leader?

   b. How does this leader's leadership styles compare with the leader you characterized?

    c. What are three characteristics that you perceive in the health care team that contribute to and/or detract from this leader's effectiveness?

    d. What is the main attribute or characteristic this leader possesses that contributes to successful leadership? Explain your answer.

3. The feedback is estimated to require at least 300 words to adequately address these questions.

4. The feedback will be evaluated based on satisfactorily answering the four questions.

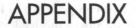

APPENDIX

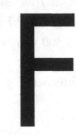

LEADING BY TEACHING STUDENT PRESENTATION

The Leading by Teaching Student Presentation engages the student in exploring a teaching exercise that reflects the practice of personal leadership strategies.

LEARNING OBJECTIVE

After completion of this assignment, the student will be able to apply leadership strategies during teaching opportunities.

Prerequisite knowledge: The student should have reviewed at least Chapters 1 through 6 and 11 prior to this activity.

LEARNER CONTENT AND DESIGN

The leading by teaching student presentation requires the student to exercise skills in leadership in the framework of teaching others. The student creates an instructional media presentation (e.g., PowerPoint or other media) to explore a topic that has general appeal in health care: *The Virtue of Personal Health Care*. The student is invited to identify a setting suitable to the student's potential leadership role (e.g., patient education setting, community health setting, academic setting, or peer professional development setting). In presenting the topic as a *virtue*, the student must explore the issues of character and values in the presentation. This assignment encourages the student to utilize leadership strategies in teaching about this topic to keep the audience engaged.

This assignment can be conducted in a classroom setting that offers live student presentations to be given, but here it is presented as an online learning management systems (LMS) assignment. Either option promotes interaction between student peers as they each share their presentations with one another.

In this LMS format, the student posts the assignment for viewing and critique by student peers. A second assignment invites peers to share their feedback with the student–presenter on both the topic and the leadership strategies exercised. The focus of the feedback activity is to engage the student in learning about personal health care virtues as well as assessing the effectiveness of leadership strategies used in the delivery of this information by his or her peers.

OPTIONAL MODIFICATIONS

1. In selected, mature learner settings, sharing this assignment among peers for the benefit of peer feedback may be valuable.

LEADING BY TEACHING STUDENT PRESENTATION ASSIGNMENT

1. **Select an educational setting in your vicinity that offers access to a population of "learners."** This could be a patient care setting (providing patient education), a community setting (providing community health education), an academic setting (providing formal instruction in a classroom), or a peer professional development setting (continuing professional education in a work setting).

2. **Develop and give a presentation on the topic of *the virtue of personal health care*.** This should be developed as if addressed to the proposed population of learners, but will be posted on the Discussion Board for your peers and instructor to view. The topic should encompass aspects of general health and hygiene, including a discussion of the intrinsic value of health as a principle of personal excellence.

3. **Elements that must be addressed in your presentation:**

   a. What is the virtue of personal health care?

   b. What is the opposite of this virtue?

   c. Use a well-known figure from history or current times to illustrate the virtue of personal health care.

   d. Describe the steps to achieve this virtue.

4. **Suggestions for aspects of this topic to address in your presentation include:**

   a. Being true to yourself

   b. Self-care emotionally, psychologically, physically, and spiritually

   c. Seeking the highest standard of health and well-being

   d. Promotion of individual and collective well-being

   e. Other aspects of personal health care at its best

5. **Requirements of the presentation**

   a. All elements of topic described in 3 above are addressed.

   b. Presentation must demonstrate leadership traits and/or behaviors described in this course.

   c. Presentation must address value dimensions anticipated in audience.

   d. The presentation length should be 15 to 20 minutes.

   e. Technical requirements (the presentation can be seen and heard) are met.

6. **Media (e.g., PowerPoint [PPT]) presentation guidelines**

   a. Assemble 15 to 30 PPT slides

   b. Maintain PPT rules of thumb:

     i. No more than five lines of text per slide

     ii. No more than five words per line

     iii. Use graphics and animations as highlights

     iv. Avoid distracting graphics

7. **Create audio recording to accompany media presentation and post**

   a. Use your computer and current PPT software to voice record for each slide (see "media" options under "insert" on PPT menu bar). Or choose another electronic audio device to record your vocal presentation, cuing the PPT slides when necessary.

   b. Presentation length should be 15 to 20 minutes.

8. On Discussion Board, post a description of:

   a. The proposed audience

   b. The leadership traits demonstrated

   c. The value dimensions addressed

   d. On the same post, attach the audio file and PPT document.

Evaluation Criteria

The presentation will be evaluated according to the following criteria:

- The four required elements are addressed in the presentation.

- The presentation demonstrates the effective use of leadership traits as addressed in this course.

- The presentation appropriately addresses the value dimensions for the proposed audience.

- The length and technical requirements of assignment are met.

FEEDBACK ASSIGNMENT

1. View and listen to at least one of your peers' presentations.

2. Provide feedback to your peer's characterization on the Discussion Board by responding to these three questions:

   a. What aspect of personal health care are you motivated to reflect on for yourself based on the presentation?

   b. What leadership traits were most effectively utilized in the presentation?

   c. What recommendations do you have to improve this instruction? Provide at least two.

3. The feedback is estimated to require at least 300 words to adequately address these questions.

4. The feedback will be evaluated based on satisfactorily answering the three questions.

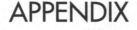

APPENDIX

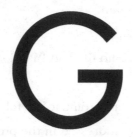

G

SELF AS LEADER
CHARACTERIZATION

The Self as Leader Characterization engages the student in reflecting on and self-assessing her or his own developing leadership qualities.

LEARNING OBJECTIVE

After completion of this assignment, the student will be able to evaluate leadership qualities, traits, and behaviors in himself or herself.

Prerequisite knowledge: The student should have reviewed at least Chapters 1 through 6 prior to this activity.

LEARNER CONTENT AND DESIGN

The characterization report requires the student to explore her or his own journey in developing as a leader, framing the evaluation by principles and concepts learned over the current study of leadership. The report concludes with self-establishing leadership goals that address the individual talents and potential opportunities as understood by the student.

Because this report encourages the student to be transparent and vulnerable, the report is not formally shared with peer learners, but is evaluated by the instructor for feedback.

OPTIONAL MODIFICATIONS

1. In selected, mature learner settings, sharing this assignment among peers for the benefit of peer feedback may be valuable.

SELF AS LEADER CHARACTERIZATION ASSIGNMENT

1. Provide a narrative report of your journey as a leader, describing the influences that have shaped your leadership, the traits or concepts of leadership that represent your leadership style, and what you anticipate is ahead as you continue to grow in leadership.

2. Please divide your report into the following three sections:

    a. Traits or qualities of leadership that represent your current leadership style.

        i. Include at least three distinct principles you've adopted as a leader.

        ii. Clearly relate these principles to concepts that have been studied in this course.

    b. Influences that have shaped your leadership over time.

        i. Include at least one story from your past that illustrates your leadership journey.

        ii. Include at least one comment from a peer or mentor of yours who offers you feedback about your leadership.

    c. Your leadership goals.

        i. Identify at least one area where you are seeking to improve your leadership skills.

        ii. Describe at least one challenge to overcome in achieving your goals.

3. The report should be limited to 1,000 to 1,500 words (2–3 pages, single-spaced).

Evaluation Criteria

The Self as Leader Characterization will be evaluated according to the following criteria:

○ **Leadership qualities:** Identified qualities give a genuine representation of leadership related to concepts in this course.

- ○ **Leadership influences:** The student's growth in leadership over time is reflected in a thoughtful description including peer/mentor feedback.

- ○ **Challenges:** The goals presented include a realistic discussion of areas for improvement, including a reasonable response to legitimate challenges.

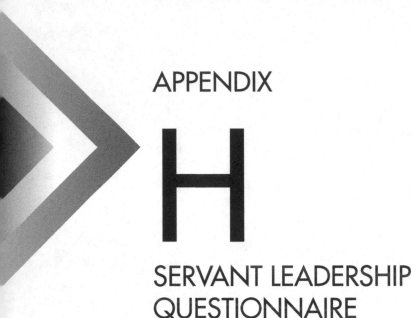

APPENDIX

H

SERVANT LEADERSHIP QUESTIONNAIRE

The Servant Leadership Questionnaire (SLQ) is designed to be administered as a self-evaluation by the leader analyzed together with results from a comparable SLQ completed by those who are familiar with the leader.

The Leader Form is administered to the leader, and the Rater Form is administered to at least two and preferably more individuals who are familiar with the leadership capacity of the leader, such as coworkers and peers, including those at a higher organizational level and those at a lower organizational level.

Scoring the SLQ

The SLQ is scored using the formula that follows (see SLQ Individual Scoring Formula). Those scores for items from the Rater Forms should be added together and that sum divided by the number of raters, resulting in the average score for each item. These averaged items associated with each factor are then added together and divided by the number of items for that factor ("4" for altruistic calling and emotional healing, "5" for the other three factors) to provide an overall score for that factor. These factor scores may then be compared to the factor scores from the Leader Form.

This comparison of the Leader Form scores with the averaged Rater Form scores determines what the leader perceives about her or his own servant leader behaviors compared to how those around the leader view his or her servant leadership.

Servant Leadership Questionnaire (SLQ)

Leader Form

My Name: _____

This questionnaire is to describe your leadership behaviors and attitudes as you perceive them. Please answer all of the questions. Please indicate how well each of the following statements describes you.

Use the following rating scale:

Not at All	Once in a While	Sometimes	Fairly Often	Frequently, If Not Always
0	1	2	3	4

_____ 1. I put others' interests ahead of my own.

_____ 2. I do everything I can to serve others.

_____ 3. I am someone to whom others will turn if they have a personal trauma.

_____ 4. I am alert to what's happening around me.

_____ 5. I offer compelling reasons to get others to do things.

_____ 6. I encourage others to dream "big dreams" about the organization.

_____ 7. I am good at anticipating the consequences of decisions.

_____ 8. I am good at helping others with their emotional issues.

_____ 9. I have great awareness of what is going on.

_____ 10. I am very persuasive.

_____ 11. I believe that the organization needs to play a moral role in society.

_____ 12. I am talented at helping others heal emotionally.

_____ 13. I am in touch with what is going on.

_____ 14. I am good at convincing others to do things.

_____ 15. I believe that our organization needs to function as a community.

_____ 16. I sacrifice my own interests to meet others' needs.

_____ 17. I can help others mend their hard feelings.

_____ 18. I am gifted when it comes to persuading others.

_____ 19. I see the organization for its potential to contribute to society.

_____ 20. I encourage others to have a community spirit in the workplace.

____21. I go above and beyond the call of duty to meet others' needs.

____22. I know what is going to happen.

____23. I am preparing the organization to make a positive difference in the future.

Source: Barbuto, J. E., & Wheeler, D. W. (2006). Scale development and construct clarification of servant leadership. *Group & Organization Management, 31*(3), 300–326. doi:10.1177/1059601106287091. Used with the author's permission.

Servant Leadership Questionnaire (SLQ)

Rater Form

Name of Leader: _____

     This questionnaire is to describe the leader behaviors and attitudes of the aforementioned individual as you perceive them. Please answer all of the questions to best describe this person. Please indicate how well each of the following statements describes this person. Please answer the questionnaire anonymously.

IMPORTANT (necessary for processing): Which best describes you?

___ I am at a higher organizational level than the person I am rating.

___ The person I am rating is at my organizational level.

___ I am at a lower organizational level than the person I am rating.

___ I do not wish my organizational level to be known.

Use the following rating scale:

Not at All	Once in a While	Sometimes	Fairly Often	Frequently, If Not Always
0	1	2	3	4

_____1. This person puts my interests ahead of his or her own.

_____2. This person does everything he or she can to serve me.

_____3. This person is one to whom I would turn if I had a personal trauma.

_____4. This person seems alert to what's happening.

_____5. This person offers compelling reasons to get me to do things.

_____6. This person encourages me to dream "big dreams" about the organization.

_____7. This person is good at anticipating the consequences of decisions.

_____8. This person is good at helping me with my emotional issues.

_____9. This person has great awareness of what is going on.

____10. This person is very persuasive.

____11. This person believes that the organization needs to play a moral role in society.

_____12. This person is talented at helping me to heal emotionally.

_____13. This person seems very in touch with what is going on.

_____14. This person is good at convincing me to do things.

_____15. This person believes that our organization needs to function as a community.

_____16. This person sacrifices his or her own interests to meet my needs.

_____17. This person is one who could help me mend my hard feelings.

_____18. This person is gifted when it comes to persuading me.

_____19. This person sees the organization for its potential to contribute to society.

_____20. This person encourages me to have a community spirit in the workplace.

_____21. This person goes above and beyond the call of duty to meet my needs.

_____22. This person seems to know what's going to happen.

_____23. This person is preparing the organization to make a positive difference in the future.

SLQ Items and SL Factors

Altruistic Calling ($\alpha \cdot .82$)

01 This person puts my best interests ahead of his/her own.

02 This person does everything he/she can to serve me.

16 This person sacrifices his/her own interests to meet my needs.

21 This person goes above and beyond the call of duty to meet my needs.

Emotional Healing ($\alpha \cdot .91$)

03 This person is one to whom I would turn if I had a personal trauma.

08 This person is good at helping me with my emotional issues.

12 This person is talented at helping me to heal emotionally.

17 This person is one who could help me mend my hard feelings.

Wisdom ($\alpha \cdot .92$)

04 This person seems alert to what's happening.

07 This person is good at anticipating the consequences of decisions.

09 This person has great awareness of what is going on.

13 This person seems very in touch with what is going on.

26 This person seems to know what is going to happen.

Persuasive Mapping ($\alpha \cdot .87$)

05 This person offers compelling reasons to get me to do things.

06 This person encourages me to dream "big dreams" about the organization.

10 This person is very persuasive.

14 This person is good at convincing me to do things.

18 This person is gifted when it comes to persuading me.

Organizational Stewardship ($\alpha \cdot .89$)

11 This person believes that the organization needs to play a moral role in society.

15 This person believes that our organization needs to function as a community.

19 This person sees the organization for its potential to contribute to society.

20 This person encourages me to have a community spirit in the workplace.

23 This person is preparing the organization to make a positive difference in the future.

SLQ Individual Scoring Formula

Altruistic Calling:	1)____,	2)____,	16)____,	21)____		= _____	(Sum)
Emotional Healing:	3)____,	8)____,	12)____,	17)____		= _____	(Sum)
Wisdom:	4)____,	7)____,	9)____,	13)____	26)____	= _____	(Sum)
Persuasive Mapping:	5)____,	6)____,	10)____,	14)____	18)____	= _____	(Sum)
Organizational:							
Stewardship:	11)____,	15)____,	19)____,	20)____	23)____	= _____	(Sum)

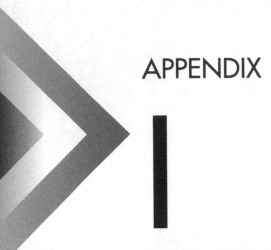

APPENDIX

I

ADAPTIVE LEADERSHIP QUESTIONNAIRE

This questionnaire is composed of 30 items. When administered as directed, it provides a 360-degree, or multirater, feedback about an individual's adaptive leadership by assessing six dimensions: get on the balcony, identify the adaptive challenge, regulate distress, maintain disciplined attention, give the work back to people, and protect leadership voices from below.

The results will provide information on how the individual views herself/himself and how others view the individual on these six dimensions of adaptive leadership.

The questionnaire is intended for practical applications. It is not designed for research purposes. For research purposes, the psychometric properties of the questionnaire (i.e., reliability and validity) would need to be established.

Adaptive leadership is a complex process, and taking this questionnaire will guide understanding of the theory of adaptive leadership as well as an individual's own style of adaptive leadership.

Order Detail ID: 70322961

Leadership: Theory and Practice by Northouse, Peter Guy (2016). Reproduced with permission of SAGE Publications, Inc. in the format Republish in a book via Copyright Clearance Center.

Adaptive Leadership Questionnaire (ALQ)

My Name: _____

Instructions: This questionnaire contains items that assess different dimensions of adaptive leadership and will be completed by you and others who know you (coworkers, friends, members of a group to which you belong).

1. Make five copies of this questionnaire.

2. Fill out the assessment about yourself; where you see the phrase "this leader," replace it with "I" or "me."

3. Have each of five individuals indicate the degree to which they agree with each of the 30 statements that follow regarding your leadership by circling the number from the scale that they believe most accurately characterizes their response to the statement. There are no right or wrong responses.

Use the following rating scale:

Strongly disagree	Disagree	Neutral	Agree	Strongly agree
1	2	3	4	5

1. When difficulties emerge in our organization, this leader is good at stepping back and assessing the dynamics of the people involved.

2. When events trigger strong emotional responses among employees, this leader uses his/her authority as a leader to resolve the problem.

3. When people feel uncertain about organizational change, they trust that this leader will help them work through the difficulties.

4. In complex situations, this leader gets people to focus on the issues they are trying to avoid.

5. When employees are struggling with a decision, this leader tells them what he/she thinks they should do.

6. During times of difficult change, this leader welcomes the thoughts of group members with low status.

7. In difficult situations, this leader sometimes loses sight of the "big picture."

8. When people are struggling with a value conflict, this leader uses his or her expertise to tell them what to do.

9. When people begin to be disturbed by unresolved conflicts, this leader encourages them to address the issues.

10. During organizational change, this leader challenges people to concentrate on the "hot" topics.

11. When employees look to this leader for answers, he/she encourages them to think for themselves.

12. Listening to group members with radical ideas is valuable to this leader.

13. When this leader disagrees with someone, he/she has difficulty listening to what the other person is really saying.

14. When others are struggling with intense conflicts, this leader steps in to resolve their differences for them.

15. This leader has the emotional capacity to comfort others as they work through intense issues.

16. When people try to avoid controversial organizational issues, this leader brings these conflicts into the open.

17. This leader encourages his/her employees to take initiative in defining and solving problems.

18. This leader is open to people who bring up unusual ideas that seem to hinder the progress of the group.

19. In challenging situations, this leader likes to observe the parties involved and assess what's really going on.

20. This leader encourages people to discuss the "elephant in the room."

21. People recognize that this leader has confidence to tackle challenging problems.

22. This leader thinks it is reasonable to let people avoid confronting difficult issues.

23. When people look to this leader to solve problems, he/she enjoys providing solutions.

24. This leader has an open ear for people who don't seem to fit in with the rest of the group.

25. In a difficult situation, this leader will step out of the dispute to gain perspective on it.

26. This leader thrives on helping people find new ways of coping with organizational problems.

27. People see this leader as someone who holds steady in the storm.

28. In an effort to keep things moving forward, this leader lets people avoid issues that are troublesome.

29. When people are uncertain about what to do, this leader empowers them to decide for themselves.

30. To restore equilibrium in the organization, this leader tries to neutralize comments of out-group members.

ALQ Scoring Formula

Get on the Balcony: This score represents the degree to which you are able to step back and see the complexities and interrelated dimensions of a situation.

To arrive at this score:

Sum items 1, 19, and 25 and the reversed (R) score values for 7 and 13 (i.e., change 1 to 5, 2 to 4, 4 to 2, and 5 to 1, with 3 remaining unchanged).

1 _____ 7(R) _____ 13(R) _____ 19 _____ 25 _____ Total _____

Identify the Adaptive Challenge: This score represents the degree to which you recognize adaptive challenges and do not respond to these challenges with technical leadership.

To arrive at this score:

Sum items 16 and 20 and the reversed (R) score values for 2, 8 and 14 (i.e., change 1 to 5, 2 to 4, 4 to 2, and 5 to 1, with 3 remaining unchanged).

2(R) _____ 8(R) _____ 14(R) _____ 16 _____ 20 _____ Total _____

Regulate Distress: This score represents the degree to which you provide a safe environment in which others can tackle difficult problems and to which you are seen as confident and calm in conflict situations.

To arrive at this score:

Sum items 3, 9, 15, 21, and 27.

3 _____ 9 _____ 15 _____ 21 _____ 27 _____ Total _____

Maintain Disciplined Attention: This score represents the degree to which you get others to face challenging issues and not let them avoid difficult problems.

To arrive at this score:

Sum items 4, 10, and 26 and the reversed (R) score values for 22 and 28 (i.e., change 1 to 5, 2 to 4, 4 to 2, and 5 to 1, with 3 remaining unchanged).

4 _____ 10 _____ 22(R) _____ 26 _____ 28(R) _____ Total _____

Give the Work Back to People: This score is the degree to which you empower others to think for themselves and solve their own problems.

To arrive at this score:

Sum items 11, 17, and 29 and the reversed (R) score values for 5 and 23 (i.e., change 1 to 5, 2 to 4, 4 to 2, and 5 to 1, with 3 remaining unchanged).

5(R) _____ 11 _____ 17 _____ 23(R) _____ 29 _____ Total _____

Protect Leadership Voices From Below: This score represents the degree to which you are open and accepting of unusual or radical contributions from low-status group members.

To arrive at this score:

Sum items 6, 12, 18, and 24 and the reversed (R) score value for 30 (i.e., change 1 to 5, 2 to 4, 4 to 2, and 5 to 1, with 3 remaining unchanged).

6 _____ 12 _____ 18 _____ 24 _____ 30(R) _____ Total _____

ALQ Scoring Chart

To complete the scoring chart, enter the raters' scores and your own scores in the appropriate column on the scoring sheet below. Find the average score from your five raters, and then calculate the difference between the average and your self-rating.

	Rater 1	Rater 2	Rater 3	Rater 4	Rater 5	Average Rating	Self-Rating	Difference
Get on the Balcony								
Identify the Adaptive Challenge								
Regulate Distress								
Maintain Disciplined Attention								
Give the Work Back to the People								
Protect Leadership Voices From Below								

ALQ Scoring Interpretation

High range: A score between 21 and 25 means you are strongly inclined to exhibit this adaptive leadership behavior.

Moderately high range: A score between 16 and 20 means you moderately exhibit this adaptive leadership behavior.

Moderately low range: A score between 11 and 15 means you at times exhibit this adaptive leadership behavior.

Low range: A score between 5 and 10 means you are seldom inclined to exhibit this adaptive leadership behavior.

This questionnaire measures adaptive leadership by assessing six components of the process: get on the balcony, identify the adaptive challenge, regulate distress, maintain disciplined attention, give the work back to people, and protect leadership voices from below. By comparing your scores on each of these components, you can determine which are your stronger and which are your weaker components. The scoring chart allows you to see where your perceptions are the same as those of others and where they differ.

There are no "perfect" scores for this questionnaire. While it is confirming when others see you in the same way as you see yourself, it is also beneficial to know when they see you differently. This assessment can help you understand those dimensions of your adaptive leadership that are strong and dimensions of your adaptive leadership you may seek to improve.

INDEX

Printed in the United States
By Bookmasters